Our NHS: A celebration of 50 years

Our NHS: A celebration of 50 years

Edited by
Gordon Macpherson
Former Deputy Editor of the British Medical Journal

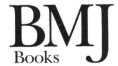

First published in 1998
by BMJ Books, BMA House, Tavistock Square,
London WC1H 9JR

British Library Cataloguing in Publication Data

A catalogue record for this book is available from the British Library

ISBN 0–7279–1289–5

Typeset by Apek Typesetters, Nailsea, Bristol
Printed and bound by Latimer Trend & Company Ltd., Plymouth

Cover image shows Beveridge, Bevan, Castle, and Clarke. Reproduced with permission from Getty Images and Rex Features.

Contents

Foreword

The UK National Health Service is unique. It is unique historically, having been conceived during the long night of bitter global conflict by a coalition government uniting faith in a pacific future with the vision bright of a land fit for heroes and it first saw the light of day in the bathetic aftermath of an exhausting victory. It is unique economically, in acceptance of collective responsibility for the health of all the people; ethically, in enshrining the principles of the Judeo-Christian and utilitarian traditions; politically, in achieving a broad consensus among the people, their government and the professions who care for them. Beveridge's blueprint for the Welfare State echoed Disraeli's priority for health as the basis for national prosperity in its essential criterion of a comprehensive national health service free to all at times of need. It was tailored to a national need and a national creed.

That dedicated midwife Aneurin Bevan anticipated teething problems but was to be proved optimistic about the cost of rearing a child whose appetite exceeded both expectations and resources. Hence it was fed hand to mouth until early adolescence when another visionary Celt of a different political hue, Enoch Powell, encouraged by the medical profession's Porritt Report, stimulated debate about its development in adult life. This led first to administrative changes and later, in successive reorganisations, to the transition from administration to management, culminating at the dangerous age of 40 in the theoretical concept of an "internal market". As we celebrate the NHS's ripe maturity a decade further on, it is time to take stock. What can we learn from the past to inspire the future?

The world has moved on. The Welfare State has become the "Fare well" state, in which medical advances have contributed their mead to "adding years to life and life to years" but in which widening inequalities not only challenge our collective conscience but too often deprive those in greatest need. Then there is the mismatch between the commendable *Health of the Nation* philosophy and strategy, with its emphasis on intersectoral collaboration, participation by the people, health promotion, and disease prevention on the one hand, and the spectre of "winners and losers" in a health market, on the other.

As the NHS enters the second half of its first century, a fresh consensus has emerged; that function must dictate structure, not the converse.

Pragmatism – tutored by trauma – must replace ideology. Need – relative, clinical need – must prevail over capricious demand and outcomes over output. Cost effectiveness must supersede cost efficiency. What matters is that patients come out of the system vertically, not horizontally. Evidence of benefit to the patient is the new *leitmotif* and quality the watchword. There is a hunger for healing, not only literally in the provision of patient care but in relationships between all the players in the field – ministers, health authorities, trusts, staff, and the patients whom we serve. New alliances are being formed in recognition of the imperative of teamwork at all levels. There is universal agreement that the NHS vehicle needs a clearer destination, regular maintenance, more fuel in the tank, and better education and training for its drivers. Research is crucial to improve every element of the system. Debate will predictably intensify about alternative sources of funding, although direct taxation is demonstrably the fairest and friendliest method. Prioritisation will continue to do battle with rationing; occasionally, especially when disasters strike less fortunate lands, we will thank a provident society for the benefits of our NHS, however imperfect it may be.

Inevitably in a BMA publication on health care, the doctors take centrestage and the spotlight falls mercilessly on them, but as the story unfolds the other actors enter timorously from the wings. A distinguished company of authors, themselves players, producers and programme directors, has been assembled to review and, where appropriate, to preview events against the background of the theatre in which the drama of life and death unendingly unfolds. There is an unspoken implicit assumption that the curtain is not about to fall upon the stage of the NHS. Here the players neither strut nor fret their hours upon the stage; their tale signifies everything that matters about an institution which is very much alive and which could well remain so in whatever guise, even to the "last syllable of recorded time".

A. W. MACARA
Chairman of Council
British Medical Association

Introduction

A flavour of the NHS

Aneurin Bevan launched our National Health Service on 5 July 1948. I use the pronoun deliberately because Britons are possessive about the NHS in a way that they are not about other state funded services. Nicholas Timmins in his excellent analysis of the welfare state, *The Five Giants,*[1] describes the "Appointed Day" of 5 July as "by any standards one of the great days of British history". Certainly for patients - the NHS's raison d'être - the service has been a success, though public satisfaction has fallen over the past decade or so. Doctors, too, despite some initial hostility, soon came to support the NHS as enthusiastically as their patients. Indeed, at the turn of this decade the British Medical Association - doctors' largest professional organisation - was perhaps the most vociferous of the critics who feared that the proposed internal market for the NHS would undermine the service's basic principle: comprehensive, state funded medical care for all who need it.

The BMA is marking the 50th anniversary of the NHS with this volume of invited personal perspectives from individuals who have worked in or been closely associated with the service. The association is grateful to all contributors for their cooperation (see page 00 for their CVs), and I feel privileged to have been asked to edit this anniversary publication.

Setting the scene

The book is not a history of the NHS's first five decades - others have written that[2,3] -nor does it attempt to cover all the successes, failures and controversies of this enormous, complex and constantly evolving organisation. The aim has been to give readers a genuine flavour of the NHS, and the scene is set by four distinguished doctors.

- Lord Walton, an eminent neurologist and a past president of the General Medical Council, provides a panorama of the past 50 years.

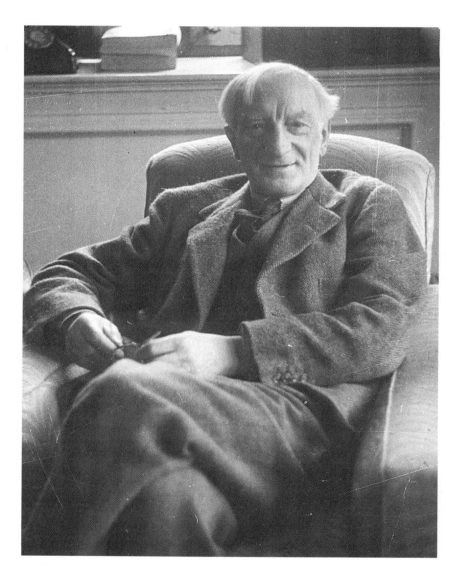

William (later Lord) Beveridge. His 1942 report *Social Insurance and Allied Services*, which laid the groundwork for Britain's postwar welfare state, was an immediate best seller. Reproduced with permission from Getty Images.

- Sir George Godber, a Ministry of Health doctor in the 1940s who rose to become an admirable and effective Chief Medical Officer, recounts the planning and launch of the health service.
- Sir Douglas Black, former professor of medicine and joint author of the influential sociomedical report, *Inequalities in Health*, sets the NHS in the context of people's social circumstances.
- Lord Owen, a one time Minister for Health and subsequently Foreign Secretary, examines three noted stand-offs between governments and the medical profession, illustrating - in my view - that, like it or not, politics and medicine are inextricably entwined in a state funded, centrally controlled service.

Other contributors tell what it has been like working in the NHS, offer views on its management and provision of resources, trace the fluctuating fortunes of the public health sector and examine the symbiotic relations between the NHS, medical education and research. There are also observations on the BMA's close and sometimes fractious relations with successive governments. The authors were also invited to provide a succinct forecast on where the NHS should or might be heading. Despite the recent organisational upheavals, the perennial conflicts over the provision of resources and much publicised reports of the increasing pressures on hospitals and family practitioner and community care services, most of the comments on the future are positive.

A mainly medical perspective

Most of the perspectives on the NHS that follow are written by doctors, and this volume concentrates primarily on the medical services*. Under 10% of the NHS's one million staff are doctors and they are dependent on the many skilled and supporting staff to provide patients with effective medical care. Nevertheless, doctors' presence at the medical heart of the NHS and the influence they have wielded at all levels from Whitehall to the organisation of curative and preventive medicine in hospital and general practice give their views a special provenance.

The culture of the NHS in which doctors were for long a dominant force has been transformed during the past 15 years. In 1998 the powerful voices of business executives, managers, accountants, health economists and other professionals compete with those of doctors. Indeed, since the internal market was introduced in 1991 managers have increasingly dominated the running of the health service in hospitals. General practitioners, however, are still masters of their local domains. Their independent contractor status, retained after a battle with Aneurin Bevan in the run up to the NHS, has

* The contributions were written in the latter half of 1997 and some comments may have been overtaken by subsequent events.

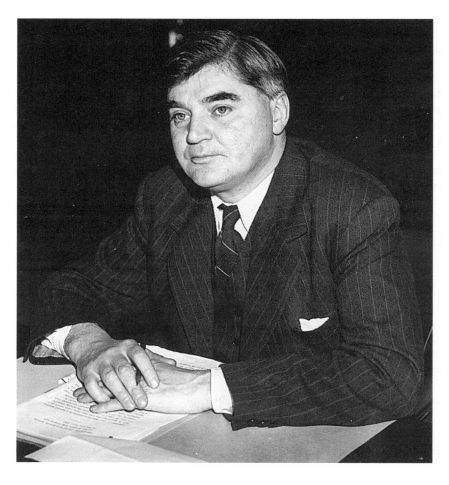

Aneurin Bevan, Minister of Health in the postwar Labour Government from 1945 to 1951. was the political architect of the National Health Service, initiating the necessary legislation and launching the service on 5 July 1948. Reproduction with permission from Getty Images.

served them and their patients well over the years. Family doctors are still responsible for contracting for 24 hour general medical care to their patients, and as leaders of primary health care teams – most now based in well equipped, modern premises – they cope with over 90% of patients' illnesses. The GPs' position as gatekeepers to the specialist services has contributed to the cost effectiveness of the NHS. Furthermore, their independence has also enabled them to speak up for their patients, a privilege that, sadly, staff in the hospital service find hard to exercise in today's business oriented culture.

Nationwide network of specialist care

One aspect of the service that would delight Bevan were he to return to the NHS in 1998 is the fulfilment of his aim for a nationwide network of good quality specialist services. Given that he put the hospital sector together from a collection of over 3,000 voluntary and municipal hospitals of widely varying quality, this has been a signal achievement of the NHS. One caveat to this achievement has been the services for patients with mental illness or learning difficulties: these services suffered some institutional scandals and then when community services for such patients became policy, successive governments failed to provide the necessary funds to ensure acceptable standards of service.

Ironically, the hospital service's very success has led to its present predicament in which patients with non-urgent conditions may have to wait many months for treatment and even some acutely ill patients can be admitted only at the expense of the premature discharge of an existing inpatient. Translation of the spectacular advances in medical research into routine hospital procedures has contributed to the pressure on hospitals. More people need or seek these new and usually expensive treatments and despite more efficient use of beds - in paticular, by the widespread development of day surgery - the resources available cannot match the rising demand. Nor will NHS resources stretch to provide institutional care for the rising number of elderly people who need it: that intractable problem is being examined by a Royal Commission.

Perennial shortage of resources

Bevan would certainly be familiar, if not comfortable, with the NHS's perennial shortage of resources - despite a five-fold (inflation adjusted) increase in funding over 50 years. It was a problem he faced soon after the service started and eventually prompted the first of many inquiries into the NHS. The Guillebaud[4] inquiry showed, however, that the service was consuming a falling share of the Gross National Product, a finding that probably saved the NHS.

The pent up demand from patients for treatment in the service's early years, the need to modernise outdated facilities, and unrealistic financial forecasts all contributed to the early funding crises. Pay demands from staff – a constant cause of dispute throughout the five decades – were an added, if understandable, pressure. One result was the introduction of charges for some services, a first breach of the principle of a free service. Surprisingly perhaps, though the charges for some dental care, spectacles and medicines were steadily increased over the years, it was not until the past decade or so that further erosion of the principle occurred with the virtual privatisation of general ophthalmic services, a gradual privatisation of dental services, and the contracting out to commercial organisations of many NHS support services.

The NHS has suffered numerous official inquiries, several reorganisations and management reforms as governments struggled to improve its efficiency and contain costs. What no government has dared do is take the political risk of radical financial reform because of the widespread public support for a tax funded service. Even when introducing the 1991 internal market - a move prompted by a financial crisis in 1988 - the then Conservative Government went to great lengths to reassure the nation that it would not undermine the principle of a "free" service. Critics, including the BMA, were doubtful about this claim. But in 1998, as a Labour Government plans to modify the internal market structures, the NHS remains largely a tax based service, something that would greatly please its political founder. It would also delight Sir William Beveridge, whose watershed 1942 report proposing a postwar Welfare State was the primer for the 1946 legislation that gave Britons their National Health Service.

Finally, what do Britons feel about the NHS in the 1990s? Certainly, patients now have more effective ways of expressing their views than when the service started. Community health councils, the *Patients' Charter*, simpler and more effective complaints procedures, the health ombudsman and well publicised government targets for health have all contributed to greater openness in the NHS. Furthermore, the media has contributed significantly to informing the public about health issues and about the NHS's strengths and weaknesses. An authoritative survey in 1996 on British social attitudes[5] reported that 80% of people nominated "health as their top or second priority for additional government spending". In 1983 the figure was 60%. Dissatisfaction, however, has doubled from 25% to 50% over the same period. More encouragingly, over 75% of those surveyed were satisfied with their general practitioner. But between 1983 and 1996 satisfaction with the hospital service fell from 74% to 53%, with waiting times the main target for criticism along with fears of premature discharge of inpatients. The survey also showed that the public believed "that the NHS must be saved by extra spending, not by looking for radical savings". This is an uncompromising message for politicians and professionals in the NHS's 50th anniversary year. It is one that Aneurin Bevan would have welcomed.

Gordon Macpherson

1. Nicholas Timmins. *The Five Giants: A biography of the Welfare State* London: Harper Collins, 1995.
2. Charles Webster. Two volume official history: *The Health Services Since the War*; volume I HMSO, 1968; volume II the Stationary Office, 1996.
3. Geoffrey Rivett. *From Cradle to Grave: fifty years of the NHS* London: The King's Fund, 1998.
4. *Report of Enquiry into the Cost of the National Health Service*, Cmnd 9663, HMSO 1956.
5. Social and Community Planning Research. *British Social Attitudes: the end of Conservative values?* Ashgate Publishing, 1997.

Contributors

Sir Douglas Black, Q 1936 (St Andrews) MD, FRCP, FRCPE KE (or KESt J).

He was Consultant Physician at Manchester Royal Infirmary from 1948 to 1977 and a member of the Medical Research Council from 1966 to 1977. He was Chief Scientist at the Department of Health and Social Services from 1973 to 1977, Chairman of the Inquiry into Inequalities in Health from 1977 to 1979 and President of the Royal College of Physicians, London, from 1977 to 1983 and President of the BMA from 1984 to 1985. Past interests – body fluid, medical ethics; present interests – deprivation and health, the effects of the NHS "reforms".

Professor George Davey Smith, Q 1983 (Cambridge), BA (Hons) (Oxford), MB BChir, MA, MSc Epidemiology, MD, FFPHM.

Professor of Clinical Epidemiology at Bristol University. His main interests are in life course influences on disease in adulthood, epidemiological methodology including meta-analysis, sexually transmitted disease epidemiology and prevention, and the social construction of medical knowledge.

Professor Brian Edwards CBE, Hon FRCPath.

He worked in the NHS for 38 years before moving into the chair of Health Care Development at the University of Sheffield in 1996. From a junior post at Clatterbridge Hospital, he climbed the management ladder (York, Leeds, Hull, Mansfield, Cheshire) and emerged as the Chief Executive of two regions (Trent and West Midlands). Professor Edwards has taught and written about health matters throughout his career, which includes extensive overseas experience.

Dr Arnold Elliott OBE, Q 1944 (Belfast) MB BCh, FRCGP.

Began work in the NHS in July 1948 and was a general practitioner in Ilford for 43 years. One-time Secretary of his local medical committee, Dr Elliott was a member of the BMA's General Medical Services Committee for 33 years and of the BMA Council for 20 years. Chaired the association's Doctors and Social Work Committee and the Community Health Committee. President, Society of Family Practitioner Committees, England and Wales, 1980. Elected member of GMC for 10 years. Member of Central Council for Education and Training Social Work for 10 years.

Dr Somerled Fergusson MBE, Q 1947 (Edinburgh) MB ChB, DFFP, FRCGP D(Obst) RCOG.

He was educated at Lochaber Senior Secondary School and Edinburgh University. A general practitioner for 40 years at Lochinver and Beauly, Dr Fergusson is the youngest foundation member of the Royal College of General Practitioners resident in Scotland. Interests - vocational training (21 trainees) and NHS organisation and management, particularly in rural areas. Hobbies - fishing, shooting, bowling, curling, history and archaeology.

Mr Jon Ford

Head of the BMA's Health Policy and Economic Research Unit, joined the BMA in 1976 as an economic research officer. A specialist in labour economics initially, he worked in econometrics and economic forecasting before joing the BMA.

Professor Malcolm Forsythe, Q 1961 (London) MB, BS MSc, FFPHM, FRCGP.

Attracted into medical administration by Sir John Revans, Professor Forsythe worked in three regions – Birmingham, Wessex and South East Thames, where he became Regional Medical Officer in 1972, then Regional Director of Public Health. Member of the Resource Allocation Working Party Review and board member of the Public Health Laboratory Service 1976–1995. He has had a longstanding concern for doctors' health and is currently the chairman of the General Medical Council's Working Party on performance assessment in public health medicine.

Dr Ruth Gilbert, Q 1982 (Sheffield) MB ChB, MSc Epidemiology, MD, FRCPCH.

Trained in paediatrics, Dr Gilbert is a Senior Lecturer in Clinical Epidemiology. Her research interests include cot death, screening in pregnancy and childhood, and the application of epidemiological research and methods to decision making in health care. She is director of the Centre for Evidence Based Child Health.

Dr Alan Gilmour CVO, CBE, Q 1956 (London) MB BS, FRCGP, LMSSA.

One-time NHS general practitioner then BMA Deputy Secretary, Head of Hospitals Division and Joint Consultants Committee secretariat; Director of the National Society for the Prevention of Cruelty to Children from 1979 to 1989.

Sir George Godber KCB, Q 1933 (Oxford), DM, FRCP, FFPHM.

Educated at Bedford School, New College, Oxford, London Hospital and London School of Hygiene, Sir George worked for two years in junior hospital posts, two years in Surrey County posts and 34 years in the Ministry of Health and the DHSS. A junior member of Ministry of Health planning team for the NHS, he spent ten years as Deputy Chief Medical Officer and 13 as Chief Medical Officer at the Ministry. Hospital surveyor for North Midlands with Leonard Parsons 1943, Sir George was continuously involved with central planning of the NHS from 1944 and its implementation until retirement in 1973. He led 13 successive British delegations to the World Health Assembly and was a member of its Executive Board for ten years.

Professor Chris Ham, MPhil, PhD, BA.

Professor of Health Policy and Management at the University of Birmingham and Director of the University's Health Services Management Centre. Graduating in 1972 from the University of Kent, he started his career in the NHS in 1975 when he was appointed as a research assistant at the Nuffield Centre for Health Services Studies at the University of Leeds. Since then he has held posts at the University of Bristol and the King's Fund. He joined the University of Birmingham in 1992. Professor Ham has published widely on health policy and health services research, his particular interests being the politics of health care and health care reform. He has worked in a range of countries advising politicians and civil servants. Within the UK he has been an advisor to the Audit Commission, the National Audit Office, the House of Commons Health Committee, and politicians of all parties.

Dr John Havard CBE, Q 1949 (Cambridge) MA, MD, LLM, FRCP, Hon FRCGP, Barrister-at-Law (Middle Temple).

Educated at Malvern College, Jesus College, Cambridge and Middlesex Hospital Medical School, Dr Havard was a principal in general practice for six years and secretary, East Suffolk Local Medical Committee, before joining BMA staff in1958. Served as secretary of all the association's craft committees and as Secretary of the BMA from 1980 to 1989. BMA Gold Medallist. President, British Academy Forensic Sciences 1984. Dr Havard is author of many medicolegal publications including *Detection of Secret Homicide* (Cambridge Studies in Criminology). Currently Honorary Secretary, Commonwealth Medical Association.

Professor Jack Howell CBE, Q 1950 (London) BSc, MB BS, PhD, DSc (Hon), FRCP, FACP (Hon).

After clinical academic posts in London and Manchester, Professor Howell was appointed to the Foundation Chair of Medicine at the new medical school in Southampton in 1969 and was Dean from 1978 to 1983. For the past 14 or so years he has chaired the Southampton and S.W. Hants Health Authority. President of the BMA from 1989 to 1990 and chairman of its Board of Science and Education from 1991 to 1998.

Sir Donald Irvine, Q 1958 (Durham) MB BS, MD, FRCGP.

Principal in general practice, Ashington, Northumberland from 1960 to 1996. A regional adviser in general medicine, Sir Donald was Chairman of Council of the Royal College of General Practitioners from 1982 to 1985, having previously been its Honorary Secretary from 1972 to 1978. He became a member of the General Medical Council in 1979 and in 1996 was the first GP to be elected its president. In 1990 he became a member of the Audit Commission. Sir Donald has taken a special interest in vocational training, audit and quality in general practice and has written widely on these subjects. He has been a visiting professor at American and Australian universities. His hobbies include bird watching, gardening and walking.

Dr Abdul Jaleel, Q 1963 (Punjab, Pakistan) MB BS, FRCP (Edinburgh), DTM&H.

Dr Abdul Jaleel was born in the Punjab and graduated from King Edward's Medical College, Lahore. He served in the NHS from 1963 until his retirement in 1995. From 1972 to 1995 he was consultant rheumatologist in Darlington. He chaired both the Local Consultants Committee of the BMA and the Medical Advisory Committee in the Northern Region for several years. Dr Jaleel, a Fellow of the BMA, served on the BMA's Central Consultants and Specialists Committee for several years, retiring in 1996.

Professor Rudolf Klein, MA (Oxford).

Born 1930. After taking a degree in modern history at Oxford, he spent 20 years with the London *Evening Standard* and *The Observer*. Switching to an academic career, he became Professor of Social Policy at the University of Bath in 1978. Also a Professorial Fellow of the King's Fund Policy Institute,

Professor Klein is the author of books on health care including *The New Politics of the NHS* (1995) and *Managing Scarcity* (with Patricia Day and Sharon Redmayne, 1996); he has written extensively for the *British Medical Journal*.

Dr Stephen Lock CBE, Q 1953 (Cambridge) MD, FRCP, FACP.

He was born in 1929 and trained at Cambridge University and St Bartholomew's Hospital Medical School. After house physician posts and national service in the Royal Air Force, he worked in clinical haematology for ten years before becoming full-time assistant editor of the *British Medical Journal*. He was appointed editor in 1975 and his interests focused on teaching medical writing, peer review, and research fraud, producing books on all three as well as several others. He was Founder President of the European Science Editors Association and of the Vancouver Group (the International Committee of Medical Journal Editors). He was awarded the Gold Medal of the British Medical Association, the Meritorious Award of the (US) Council of Biological Editors, and the CBE. In retirement, he has held a research associate post at the Wellcome Institute for the History of Medicine, London, and is also Editor in Chief of the forthcoming new edition of the *Oxford Companion to Medicine*.

Dr John Marks, Q 1949 (Edinburgh) MD, FRCGP, D(Obst) RCOG.

After house appointments (1948–49) and service in the RAMC (1949–51), he became a trainee and assistant in general practice in 1952. Dr Marks was principal in a group practice at Borehamwood from 1954 to 1989, chairing both the Hertfordshire Local Medical Committee and Executive Council. An active medicopolitician, he was Deputy Chairman of the BMA's General Medical Services Committee from 1974 to 1978, Chairman of the Representative Body from 1981 to 1984 and Chairman of Council from 1984 to 1990. Dr Marks has also been a member of the General Medical Council.

Dr Graeme McDonald, Q 1981 (Belfast) MB BCh, BAO, MRCPsych.

Dr McDonald was appointed consultant psychiatrist to Knockbracken Healthcare Park and the Royal Victoria Hospital in Belfast in1990. His catchment area is West Belfast. As a junior doctor he led the BMA's Junior Doctors' Committee from 1988 to 1990 and was closely involved in negotiations securing the New Deal on hours of work and Achieving a Balance on medical manpower planning. He is married to an inner city general practitioner, Linda Knox, and has four children. Presently Clinical Director for Mental Health for North and West Belfast Community Trust, Dr McDonald is Regional Adviser in Psychiatry for the Northern Ireland Council for Postgraduate Medical and Dental Education.

The Rt Hon The Lord Owen CH, Q 1963 (Cambridge) BA, MB BChir, MA.

Lord Owen was European Mediator in the former Yugoslavia from 1992 to 1995. He led the Social Democratic Party between 1983 and 1990. A former Foreign Secretary, Minister of Health and Minister for the Navy, he now chairs Middlesex Holdings plc, is a director of Abbott Laboratories Inc and Coats Viyella plc, and is Chancellor of Liverpool University.

Ms Melanie Phillips BA (Oxford).

Ms Phillips is a columnist on *The Observer* who writes about social policy and political culture. Her book *All Must Have Prizes* is a polemical account of Britain's education crisis and moral confusion.

Mr Peter Plumley, Q 1952 (Cambridge) MA, MB BChir, FRCS, MChir.

Educated at Caius College, Cambridge and the Middlesex Hospital, he was a registrar and senior surgical registrar at the Middlesex Hospital from 1961 to 1967. Appointed consultant general surgeon at the Royal East Sussex Hospital, Hastings, in 1967, he later chaired various hospital and regional committees, retiring in 1991. After retirement he became a member and then chairman of the local Community Health Council.

Professor Ray Robinson, BA, MSc (Econ).

He is Professor of Health Policy and Director of the Institute for Health Policy Studies at the University of Southampton and before joining the Institute in 1993, he was Deputy Director of the King's Fund Institute. Earlier in his career he had been a reader in economics at the University of Sussex and an economist in H.M. Treasury.

Dame Rosemary Rue CBE, Q 1951 (London and Oxford) FRCP, FFPHM, FRCPsych.

General practitioner from 1952 to 1958, and public health service from 1958 to 1965. She entered the hospital service in 1965 and became Senior Administrative Medical Officer for the Oxford Regional Hospital Board in 1971. Dame Rosemary was President of the Faculty of Community Medicine from 1986 to 1989 and of the British Medical Association from 1990 to 1991. She is a Past President of the Medical Women's Federation. Her publications include papers on general practice, women in medicine, community hospitals and health services.

Mr James Stoddart BA (Hons) (Cantab).

He started his medical career as a preclinical student at King's College, Cambridge, in October 1992. In his third preclinical year he was selected to go on a new course entitled 'Disease, Society and Sexuality' which used HIV and AIDS as a model to look at many aspects of the disease state, mostly through experiential learning. Starting his clinical course at Green College, Oxford, in September 1995, Mr Stoddart should be qualifying in July 1998. He is the BMA student representative for Oxford and enjoys contributing to the medical student magazine, drama and crosscountry running. His career plans are as yet undecided.

Professor Owen Wade CBE, Q 1945 (Cambridge and University College Hospital) MA, MB BChir, MD FRCP.

Worked in the Pneumoconiosis Unit of the Medical Research Council. Professor of Therapeutics and Pharmacology at Belfast and then Birmingham, he served as a member of the Committee on Safety of Drugs and of the Medicines Commission. Professor Wade chaired the committee that produced the present format of the *British National Formulary*.

The Lord Walton of Detchant Kt, TD, Q 1945 (Durham), MA, MD, DSc, FRCP.

Formerly consultant neurologist to the Newcastle upon Tyne Hospitals, Lord Walton was Professor of Neurology in the University and from 1971 to 1981 Dean of Medicine. From 1983 to 1989 he was Warden of Green College, Oxford. President of the British Medical Association from 1980 to 1982, of the Royal Society of Medicine from 1984 to 1986, and the General Medical Council from 1982 to 1989, Lord Walton is presently President of the World Federation of Neurology. He chaired the House of Lords Select Committee on Medical Ethics and has also been a member of its Select Committee on Science and Technology.

Sir David Weatherall KtB, Q 1956 (Liverpool) MB ChB (Hons), MD, FRCP, FRS.

After qualification he did junior hospital posts, a period of national service in Malaya and four years at Johns Hopkins Hospital, Baltimore. Returning to Liverpool in 1965, Sir David was later appointed Professor of Haematology in 1971. In 1974 he moved to Oxford as Nuffield Professor of Clinical Medicine. In 1992 he was appointed Regius Professor of Medicine at Oxford. In 1979 he became Honorary Director of the MRC Molecular Haematology Unit and in 1989 established the Institute of Molecular Medicine at Oxford, of which he is Honorary Director. His main research interests have been in the application of molecular biology to clinical medicine, particularly the genetic disorders of haemoglobin. He was knighted in 1987, elected FRS in 1977 and a Foreign Associate of the American National Academy of Sciences in 1990. In 1992 he was elected President of the British Association for the Advancement of Science.

Dr Frank Wells, Q 1960 (London) MB BS, MRCGP, FFPM.

As a medical student he always wanted to be a general practitioner. Half of his career was spent fulfilling that ambition and Dr Wells then moved on in 1979 to new challenges as undersecretary of the BMA. Seven years later, he started a decade as Medical Director of the ABPI and is now a non-executive director of an NHS trust.

Dr David Williams, Q 1949 (Liverpool) MB ChB, FRCGP.

A principal in general practice in Wales from 1954 to 1988, Dr Williams has been provost of the North Wales Faculty of the Royal College of General Practitioners. He served on the editorial committee of the *British National Formulary* from 1974 to 1976. Chairman of the Welsh General Medical Services Committee (1975–1980) and of the BMA's Welsh Council (1979–1981), he became Deputy Chairman of the General Medical Services Committee, serving from 1980 to 1982. An active Liberal Party member, Dr Williams was three times a parliamentary candidate for the Denbigh constituency and helped to prepare the party's evidence for the Royal Commission on the NHS in 1976.

BIBLIOGRAPHIES

The following authors supplied bibliographies for their essays: Professor Malcolm Forsythe, Professor Jack Howell, Professor Rudolf Klein, Lord Owen, Professor Ray Robinson, Professor Owen Wade, Lord Walton, Sir David Weatherall, and Dr David Williams. These are available on request by writing to Dr Norman Ellis at the British Medical Association.

Acknowledgments

This book originated with an idea from Dr Vivienne Nathanson, head of the professional resources and research group of the BMA. I am indebted to Dr A W Macara, Chairman of Council of the BMA, and Dr Mac Armstrong, the Association's Secretary, for their valuable support. Dr Norman Ellis, BMA Under Secretary, and Jon Ford, Head of Health Policy and Economic Research Unit, have provided essential help, for which I am grateful. I thank Patricia Langley for her hard work helping to prepare the text and Jan Croot for research on the illustrations. Mary Banks and the BMJ Book Department have my thanks for their patient and expert support.

Finally, and most importantly, the BMA is indebted to the authors, whose willing cooperation and informative contributions have, I believe, made this volume a fitting tribute to a great national institution on its 50th anniversary.

1: 1946–1996 and all that: 50 years of the NHS*

Lord Walton of Detchant

I qualified in the Newcastle Medical School of Durham University in 1945. Hence I have witnessed the gestation of the NHS, its birth and its progress into lusty middle age. The establishment of a truly universal national service has been a major achievement, of which I am a fervent supporter.

Antecedents

Contributory national health insurance for workers (often referred to as the Lloyd George Act) was first introduced in 1911, with the Ministry of Health being set up in 1913. By 1938, 43% of the population was covered. Between 1920 and 1942 many groups and individuals put forward ideas for a national health service. 1942 was to prove a crucial year: it was then that the government-initiated Beveridge Committee reported with a radical analysis of the nation's health, social, and welfare services. This led, among other things, to publication in 1944 by the Coalition Government of a White Paper on a national health service. Meanwhile, the effective Emergency Medical Service, which from 1939 had built many hospitals across the country to deal with military and civilian casualties, showed what could be achieved by government. The BMA, however, strongly opposed the White Paper's proposals, fearing a Civil Service style, local authority-dominated salaried service. The association wanted to preserve the cherished independence of the private medical practitioner and the independent voluntary hospitals.

My first experience in medicopolitics was as President of the Medical Students' Representative Council in Newcastle and as Treasurer of the British Medical Students' Association, a body then nurtured by the BMA. Influenced, no doubt, by this link, I challenged in a public debate the

* This essay is an abbreviated version of the BMA Anniversary Lecture, delivered by the author at BMA House on 6 November 1996, the 50th anniversary of the passage of the NHS Act 1946. A full version can be obtained from Dr Norman Ellis of the BMA's secretariat.

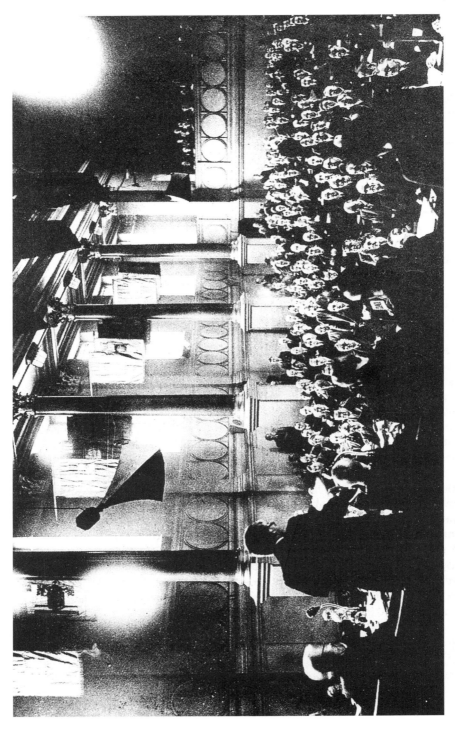

The Special Representative Meeting of the British Medical Association at its London headquarters in May 1948 when conditional cooperation in the National Health Service was agreed.

proposals of the Minister of Health, Mr Henry Willink. I saw the error of my ways when I became a house officer in a severely understaffed teaching hospital, recognising every working day the problems facing the voluntary hospitals. Newcastle's Royal Victoria Infirmary was typical: despite its substantial endowment and voluntary contributions from the local population, the hospital was in financial difficulty. Some sort of national solution seemed necessary.

Gestation: 1946–1948

When the NHS opened its doors on 5 July 1948, the country had 500,000 beds in 3105 hospitals staffed by 20,000 hospital doctors. Many of them were honorary consultants who received no remuneration from the voluntary hospitals, where they worked in the mornings, while making their income from private practice in the afternoons. Nurses numbered 150,000 but only 20,000 general practitioners served the community. Few were in partnerships and bad premises were not uncommon. When, immediately after qualification in 1946, I did a locum for a charming Northumbrian doctor to allow him to take his first holiday for five years, I could find only one elderly rubber glove and his surgery had no examination couch. While there were many dedicated and highly competent family doctors, standards were uneven and often inadequate.

The BMA, with radio doctor Charles Hill as its Secretary, fiercely opposed the proposals for an NHS, its council gravely concerned about the prospect of a salaried service and its feared effect on doctors' clinical independence. The council, led by a determined Birmingham GP, Guy Dain, was perceived as being dominated by GPs. On the hospital front, power lay with the royal colleges. Their leaders, Lord Moran and Sir Alfred Webb-Johnson, using social as well as political skills, persuaded Bevan to allow part-time consultant contracts – thus permitting NHS consultants to do private practice – and to introduce merit awards for senior and distinguished consultants. A salary for doctors working in the voluntary hospitals, which would also be state funded, was another persuasive factor. Bevan later, at a private dinner, made the oft quoted remark: "I stuffed their mouths with gold".

A proposal that GPs would be paid by a capitation fee and not a fixed salary began to turn the tide of opposition. The final vote of the BMA Council, just five weeks before the appointed day, was split 52–48, but by then so many doctors had agreed to "sign up" for the service that the battle was won and the NHS started on 5 July 1948.

The first decade

The start of the NHS saw a surge of patients, many with longstanding illnesses about which they could not previously afford to consult a doctor.

3

The service just about coped but it was a signal that the cost of the NHS was likely to be higher than the Labour government had forecast. The first year's estimate of £179 million became an actual cost of £242 million. Within a year an NHS Amendment Act was passed, which, as well as allowing private patients to be treated in health centres, imposed charges on non-UK residents and gave the government the power to levy prescription charges. In 1950 the Chancellor imposed a ceiling of £352 million on annual NHS expenditure and a year later the government introduced charges for spectacles, dentures, dental treatment, and drugs, a decision which provoked Aneurin Bevan to resign.

The Conservative Party came to power in 1952 and soon faced a potential revolt by GPs over what they saw as inadequate income. The government invited Lord Justice Dankwerts to arbitrate. He recommended a 30% pay increase. This was no doubt well deserved but it horrified the Cabinet, though it had no alternative but to agree. Increasing concern about costs prompted the government to set up the Guillebaud Inquiry, reporting in 1956. The committee discovered that whereas the NHS had consumed 3·75% of GNP in 1949, by 1953-1954 the figure had fallen to 3·25%. It therefore concluded that the service was not only underfunded but was also giving good value for money. The committee warned, however, "that the NHS administration was bogged down in a morass of committees – unnecessary committee work was an unmixed evil"; *Plus ça change!* Disputes over the pay of GPs and hospital doctors continued between the government and the profession; in 1957 the government appointed a royal commission. Reporting in 1960, it recommended a substantial pay increase and an independent body that would periodically review doctors' and dentists' remuneration.

Another sector of the NHS, the provision of drugs, had also been causing financial alarm. In an attempt to control costs the government agreed a voluntary price regulation scheme with the pharmaceutical industry in 1958.

Adolescence: 1960–1969

While governments were to continue to worry about the costs of the service, public satisfaction with the NHS continued to grow in the 1960s. Opinion polls showed that despite lengthening waiting lists for "cold" medical treatment (particularly non-urgent surgery), the public felt that they were receiving an improving standard of service, both from GPs and, when needed, from the hospitals.

In 1962, Health Minister Enoch Powell launched a hospital plan for England and Wales (and a comparable one for Scotland); the concept of the district general hospital was born and gradually old and outdated hospitals were updated or, occasionally, even replaced. More consultants were appointed in all specialties, though this expansion was painfully slow. The nursing and other health care professions had also become increasingly vocal politically. At the start of the decade my erstwhile senior colleague Henry Miller published his notable paper in *The Lancet*, "Fifty years after Flexner", criticising standards of medical education and research but above all commenting adversely upon NHS funding. In a broadcast debate with Enoch Powell, he proposed the establishment of an NHS corporation with increased funding, but his idea was not taken up.

Also in 1962, the Porritt Report, prepared by a committee broadly representative of doctors, advocated reorganisation of the NHS, with abolition of its clumsy tripartite structure. This sowed the seed for later restructuring of the service. Meanwhile, anxiety grew about standards in general practice and 1963 saw publication of the Gillie Report. This defined the primary health care team and proposed integrated community care, recommending that 146 combined health and welfare authorities should be established throughout the country. In this year, too, the Committee on the Safety of Drugs under Sir Derek Dunlop began work. Industrial turmoil, however, resurfaced and in 1965 the GPs threatened mass resignation because of what they saw as inadequate definition of their role in the primary health care team.

The BMA published the Family Doctors' Charter and started discussions with the Labour government on the future of primary care that led, in 1966, to much needed financial and structural improvements.

On the hospital front in 1966 the so-called Cogweel Reports proposed a divisional structure for hospital organisation. In teaching hospitals the divisions concerned with delivering patient services were separate from the university departments responsible for academic development, teaching, and research. A Hospital Service and Public Health Act followed in 1968, introducing standardised charges for private patients in hospital, defining the role and responsibility of university hospitals, and establishing a Medicines Commission.

The Seebohm Inquiry on social work started work in 1965 and, reporting in 1968, advocated radical restructuring of social services. It divorced the former lady almoners from their previous bases in the hospital service and set up local authority based social services which, however, continued to provide hospital social workers, in the acute and geriatric services as well as in mental health. The report enhanced social workers' training and status and was to have far reaching, though not always welcome, consequences for the NHS and the public. The Royal Commission on Medical Education (Todd Report) also appeared in 1968, making several administrative recommendations on integration between teaching hospitals' boards of governors and regional hospital boards and hospital management committees. Its proposals on other aspects of medical education were more fundamental. Prompted by forecasts of a shortage of doctors and concerns that medical school curricula and continuing education arrangements were inadequate for the needs of rapidly changing health services, the Royal Commission argued for an increase in student numbers, with new medical schools suggested and changes to how doctors were trained and kept up to date. In 1968 the government combined two big Whitehall departments into the mammoth Department of Health and Social Security, led by Richard Crossman. Also that year, in the wake of widely publicised scandals, a Hospital Advisory Service was set up to examine the care of the elderly and of the mentally ill.

The adult NHS: 1970–1979

Expansion of a consultant based service continued slowly and, mainly through the influence of the Royal College of General Practitioners (with support from the BMA's General Medical Services Committee) the standard of training of GPs and the quality of primary medical care improved steadily. Through a joint initiative of the Nuffield Provincial Hospitals Trust and the King's Fund, many postgraduate medical centres were established, often supported by public donations: postgraduate and vocational training became new buzz words.

I recall these as halcyon days in Newcastle. NHS expenditure increased steadily, new services were introduced, academic development in clinical specialties increased, in part funded by the University Grants Committee but greatly helped by the major benefactions given to the University Development Trust from individuals and industry. This facilitated many long awaited developments. Academic recognition of so-called minor and tertiary referral specialties became possible. Through the University Hospital Management Committee the university, hospital authorities and representatives of the local authorities worked as a harmonious team. At that time, with nurse and GP representation on the committee, I believe that management of the service in Newcastle reached a pinnacle of excellence never previously achieved, nor maintained since. This was also the time of exciting developments in imaging, new drugs, increasingly sophisticated technology, improved measures to relieve pain, and more effective rehabilitation. These and innumerable other advances burgeoned, with immeasurable benefits to patients but attendant steep increases in cost.

Relationships were, however, soon soured by industrial unrest. In 1970 the nurses were the first to threaten industrial action in their "raise the roof" campaign, which led to them being awarded a 22% salary increase. Inspired by McKinseys, the American management consultants, Richard Crossman produced a Green Paper on NHS reorganisation, to be followed by a consultative document in 1971. We spent many early morning and late evening committee hours considering this paper: it seemed to embody outwardly logical proposals, which we eventually adopted. How wrong we were! Sir Keith Joseph's 1972 White Paper proposed the creation of regional, area, and district health authorities along with community health councils (CHCs) to give the patients' views. This outbreak of consensus bureaucracy required representation of virtually all interested parties, a requirement that was clearly the undoing of this challenging organisational initiative. The new structure was introduced on 1 April 1974 and was a major upheaval affecting many individuals. It resulted in the creation of many planning and administrative posts which we soon recognised as unnecessary. Above all, the cornerstone principle of consensus management meant that the decision making machinery became congealed. For example, a simple proposal for a new registrar post had to be assessed by no fewer than 15 committees at national, regional, area, and hospital level before there was any chance of approval.

This administrative nonsense was further worsened by Secretary of State Barbara Castle's introduction of what she called democracy in the NHS: this increased local authority representation on health authorities. I had worked happily with many well meaning and dedicated councillors from the Newcastle City Council. With increased local authority representation and the more powerful voice of CHCs, however, we entered Alice in Wonderland country. If, say, on logical planning grounds we proposed to withdraw a specific service from a local hospital, filibustering by the councillors from that particular area meant that health authority meetings often became incapable of reaching decisions in the wider interest of the service. Consensus management, difficult at the best of times, was soon replaced by what I call decibel management (he or she who shouted the loudest won the day).

Industrial disputes irreparably damage NHS

1974 was, however, clouded by several major industrial disputes which, in my view, irreparably damaged the NHS. Firstly, the ancillary workers threatened to strike and some actually withdrew services. Secondly, the nurses threatened strike action: the government set up an inquiry, chaired by Lord Halsbury, to head off a potentially disastrous confrontation. The inquiry examined their pay and responsibilities and those of individuals working in the professions supplementary to medicine. Doctors, too, were once again in dispute, provoked by galloping national inflation. Eventually, the then Secretary of State, Barbara Castle, faced by a work to rule by many hospital doctors, awarded them a 30% pay rise. I wrote to *The Times* criticising the BMA Council for recommending industrial action, pointing out that it would inevitably hurt patients, whom doctors had been trained to serve.

In this year, too, disenchantment among junior doctors over their long hours and modest rewards came to a head. The Labour government, while refusing to grant them a well deserved big salary increase, did introduce extra duty (overtime) payments. We then had the extraordinary position of some senior registrars earning more than their consultants. Paradoxically, in Newcastle the senior registrar with most extra duty payments was a dermatologist: such anomalies were common. I believed then, and still do, that overtime payments should be anathema to a learned profession. If those problems were not enough, the Labour government, under pressure from the unions, appointed a Health Service Board to implement a progressive programme of withdrawal of pay beds from NHS hospitals (see Chapter 4). This decision contributed more to the rapid development of private practice than any other action of governments I can recall. Ludicrously, the three major Newcastle hospitals ended up with only one private bed each. As Dean of Medicine and Professor of Neurology, I regularly had patients referred from across the world. Such patients (except from the European Union) rightly had to pay the full cost of investigation and treatment. Government policy, however, meant that I was regularly compelled to refuse to accept patients from the United States and other countries as no private hospital could then offer the skilled facilities available in my NHS department. I have always believed that a public/private partnership in the NHS is to be commended. When private beds were available on many wards or NHS hospitals had private wards, consultants could be caring for both public and private patients under one roof. This saved time otherwise wasted in travelling.

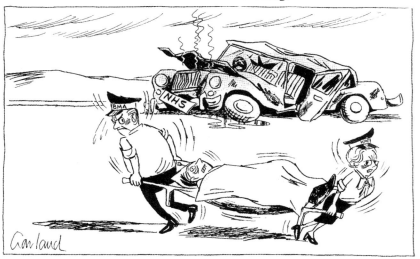

How the cartoonist Garland interpreted the arguments in 1987 between the BMA and the Conservative Government over the former's claims that the NHS was seriously underfunded. Reproduced with permission from Nicholas Garland and *The Independent*. Supplied by the Centre for the Study of Cartoons and Caricature, University of Kent, Canterbury.

Turmoil in the NHS continued and in 1976 Harold Wilson appointed a Royal Commission chaired by Sir Alec Merrison. It reported in 1979 but produced no startling recommendations. The complexities of the NHS had once again defied solution. Resources remained a constant focus of dissatisfaction – not just the overall amount allocated by the government but also their distribution. For many years the south east had received more resources per capita than the rest of England and Wales (Scotland and Northern Ireland had their own, more generous, budgets) and wide variations occurred in allocations within regions. This resulted in many areas with high morbidity being unfairly penalised. These serious anomalies led to the birth of the Resource Allocation Working Party (RAWP). It recommended substantial redistribution of resources and gradually the disparities were lessened. 1979 also saw unrest among consultants, prompted by an increasing workload. The BMA negotiated a more work sensitive contract, which also allowed all NHS consultants (even those holding wholetime contracts) to do a limited amount of private practice. Many universities soon followed suit. In that year, too, the newly elected Conservative government published its seminal document *Patients First,* recommending yet another NHS reorganisation.

The NHS in adult life: 1980–1989

The 1980s were to prove a decade of radical change. I was involved in the changes not only as a clinician and academic but also as President of the BMA. This is normally a one year appointment and in 1980, when the BMA's annual meeting was held in Newcastle (a magnificent occasion) I served as President. Unexpectedly, I carried out the duties for three years. In 1981 the President-elect, Lord Smith of Marlow, was ill and I was invited to do a second year. In 1982, the BMA's 150th anniversary, the president was His Royal Highness The Prince of Wales and on occasions I deputised for him. So, as President or Acting President I had a unique inside view of the BMA's work during the start of the Thatcher decade.

1980 saw the publication of the Black Report on inequalities in health (p 21). Set up by the Labour government, its recommendations were buried by the new Tory administration. Meanwhile, the Tories pressed ahead with another reorganisation in 1982, this one removing the area tier. The next year saw a pay review body set up for nurses and midwives and the radical Griffiths Report to streamline NHS management was published (p 37). It was to have a profound effect on how the NHS was run, with delegation,

9

executive action, and accountability its dominant themes. Consensus management was consigned to history.

In 1984 the first limited list of drugs prescribable in the NHS was imposed, despite powerful opposition from both doctors and pharmacists. The following year Project 2000 was launched: this was an ambitious and farsighted exercise designed to improve the training and career prospects of the nursing profession. In 1985 also, family practitioner committees became employing authorities, while the government maintained the hectic pace in 1986 by publishing a Green Paper on primary health care as well as the Cumberlege Report on (a related subject) neighbourhood nursing. The next year the Health Education Council, a body some criticised as being left wing, was replaced by a new Health Education Authority. In that year, too, the joint government/profession report on junior hospital doctors' prospects, *Achieving a Balance*, was published. This proposed an increase in the consultant establishment, a reduction in junior doctors' hours, and a link between the number of junior posts and projected consultant vacancies.

1988 was notable for the reversal of Richard Crossman's amalgamation of health and social security, with the DHSS split into two departments. The expected community care report – a second influential commentary by Sir Roy Griffiths - was published after delays caused by Whitehall infighting over which departments should take what responsibilities. A clinical grading structure for nurses was introduced to give clinical nurses better career prospects. However, a series of well publicised incidents highlighting the inadequacy of some clinical services, especially in neonatal intensive care, yet again prompted claims of inadequate funding. Public and politicians became alarmed and the high profile publicity persuaded the Prime Minister to announce, during an interview on the BBC *Panorama* programme, a fundamental review of the NHS.

The NHS in middle age

Mrs Thatcher set up a small policy review group and, eschewing representation of or advice from existing medical bodies such as the BMA and royal colleges, the government published the White Paper *Working for Patients*. This proposed an internal market through which contracting of clinical services between NHS providers (hospitals) and purchasers (health authorities and some GPs) would be introduced. "Money would follow the patient," ministers claimed and competition between different NHS hospitals would thus, they argued, give better value for money. An NHS Management Executive acted as a conduit and a buffer between Whitehall and the NHS and the White Paper's proposals were embodied in the NHS and Community Care Bill. This legislation reconstituted the RHAs, the DHAs, and the special health authorities and converted family practitioner committees into family health service authorities accountable to the RHAs. I and many other crossbench peers, and indeed some from all parties in the House of Lords, criticised many clauses, not least those relating to locally negotiated pay settlement. We achieved relatively little but were at least successful in persuading the government to accept a university voice on health authorities on the grounds that research and the education of health professionals was of crucial importance.

In 1991, following a report of the House of Lords Select Committee on Science and Technology, a Director of Research and Development was appointed in the NHS, followed in 1992 by the appointment of regional directors funded by a set percentage of the NHS budget. In 1991 two key elements of the market NHS were launched: 57 first wave NHS trusts and 306 fundholding GPs. The *Patient's Charter* was also published, embodying many important principles on patients' rights. These, however, have proved difficult to implement, financial restraints being among the many reasons. In 1992 a government report on the health of the nation defined priority areas for investment in the NHS and the Tomlinson Report on the future of London's hospitals was published. Unsurprisingly, this engendered much controversy, which has persisted, prompting the new Labour government in 1997 to launch yet another review.

By 1994, 419 NHS trusts, representing 96% of hospital and community health funding in the NHS, had been set up, while the number of GP fundholders had risen to 9000. But burgeoning bureaucracy provoked great criticism and RHAs were first reorganised and then in 1996 abolished, being replaced by regional offices of the NHS Executive.

Pluses and minuses in the market style NHS

The restructured NHS launched in 1991 has had a bumpy ride but as I write in 1997, the service contains pluses, as well as minuses. Firstly, my perception of the benefits.

- The NHS still gives excellent value for money and its emergency care is as good as anywhere in the world.
- GPs' gatekeeping functions cut the costs of hospital referrals.
- All health professionals are more aware of costs.
- The quality of general practice has improved immeasurably, with those GPs who are fundholders able to purchase appropriate care for the patients.

11

- Medical audit, quality control, and evidence based medicine are improving standards of care throughout the NHS.
- The community care programme has great potential, though as yet unfulfilled.
- The number of consultants has risen.
- Developments in vocational and postgraduate training are raising standards of care.
- Collaboration among health professionals is improving, as is co-operation between hospital, primary and community care.
- Preventive medicine is being given a higher priority, long overdue.

As to the NHS's principal failings, here is my list.

- By international standards the NHS is underfunded, a condition confirmed by the struggle that trusts and health authorities face to keep within their budgets.
- In many areas unrealistic efficiency savings demanded by governments are creating severe strains on staff and facilities.
- Though the NHS has received annual above-inflation funding increases, these take insufficient account of the fact that the costs of medical services worldwide rise faster than the national inflation indices.
- The purchaser/provider split generated a massive increase (over 130%) in the number of administrative posts.
- Management and planning are fragmented because of competition between trusts.
- The quality of management varies unacceptably and some managers do not understand the workings of secondary and tertiary referrals for patients requiring specialist care.
- A fall in the number of tertiary referrals has undermined high skill tertiary centres of care, cut the quality of patient care, and affected the training of specialist staff.
- The pressure from managers on clinicians and academics is threatening standards of teaching and research, thus endangering the future quality of care and the ability of the NHS to keep up to date.
- The consequences for academic medicine of inadequately rewarded posts, a rising NHS clinical workload, and the shift of resources from hospital to community care are grave; 57 clinical professorial posts were vacant in 1996.
- The pressures on NHS and academic consultants are undermining professional satisfaction and provoking many consultants to retire well before 65.
- Early retirements from general practice are also rising while recruitment is falling, the prime reasons being heavy workloads and diminishing professional satisfaction.

12

The future

- No country can afford a publicly funded comprehensive health service to meet all its citizens' demands.
- Financial pressures will worsen because of demographic changes, medical advances, and rising public expectation.
- A publicly acceptable machinery for deciding national and local priorities should be evolved.
- An informed public might well accept a hypothecated, index linked health tax as well as a sharp rise in tax on health damaging activities such as smoking and drinking; these would be preferable to widening direct charges for services.
- More effective health education and preventive health measures are essential.
- The public/private mix of health care should continue and be developed, with NHS hospitals providing more private facilities, but the private finance initiative will be of marginal help in meeting the NHS's substantial capital requirements.
- The public's profound support for the NHS could be tapped with more determined voluntary fund raising, including a health service lottery.
- Further structural reform of the NHS will hinder, not help, its development.

In conclusion, without some radical initiatives to find additional sources of funding, rescue academic clinical medicine, improve deteriorating staff morale, stem the flow of premature retirements, and improve recruitment to general practice, nursing, and the other health care professions, I fear that our beloved NHS, to which I have devoted much of my professional lifetime, will be in danger of foundering.

2: The origin and the first 25 years: a view from the centre

Sir George Godber

Public provision for health care in Britain before 1948 was a patchwork of ill co-ordinated support, where private arrangements were insufficient. The hospital services had been largely charitable, with a background of Poor Law provision for the destitute and local authority systems for communicable disease control and care of the mentally ill. Fortunately, general medical practice had been supported by nearly 30 years of National Health Insurance and before that, patchily, by the sick club system. Preventive services of a limited kind had developed in this century for maternal and child health and school health. Neither the health professions nor the general public could be content with services so ill organised at a time when scientific progress in health care was continuously accelerating and co-ordination, with secure funding, was a necessity.

Between the wars, progress was made through a succession of changes in the law requiring action by local authorities. Bodies such as the British Hospital Association as well as the professional associations in medicine, nursing, midwifery, and dentistry produced proposals for action. World War II merely accelerated a process most of us then saw as inevitable, even if we differed over its details. The Emergency Medical Services of the war were organised on a regional basis. Even before this, the Nuffield Trust had promoted a survey of hospitals in Buckinghamshire, Berkshire, and Oxfordshire which was the forerunner of the complete review of British hospitals undertaken in 1943 by 11 teams of two or three, mainly medical, surveyors, of whom the writer was one. By then, Beveridge, in his report on Britain's welfare services, had assumed that a comprehensive health service would be organised and centrally funded and the surveyors assumed that this would happen.

1944 White Paper

A plan for England was formulated using regional planning and county and borough local support systems in a White Paper published by the wartime Coalition Government in 1944. Negotiation then began with the professions and existing hospital and local government organisations. Over the next year we stumbled toward a complex and discouraging system for hospital care, a rather more coherent primary care system for employed people, and a wider programme of community prevention and care. In 1945, Aneurin Bevan, the new Labour Minister for Health, radically changed this scene in four respects. He decided upon:

• a national takeover of all hospitals not run for profit;
• a service to be available without charge to all;
• the end of sale and purchase of medical practices;
• funding mainly from central taxation, with only a small contribution from National Insurance.

To this junior member of the planning team in the Ministry of Health, these changes brought tremendous relief.

The appointed day for the start of the NHS was 5 July 1948. That left less than two years to organise the administrative framework and I vividly recall the pressure of work on all concerned. The hospital authorities – 13 regions (later 14) in England and Wales and the five under the parallel act for Scotland – had to be appointed after local consultation and separate boards of governors were set up for teaching hospitals. The regions had to recruit their own staffs, learn about their own resources and then appoint management committees for the local groups of hospitals to be ready to take charge within a very short time. The first hospital board meeting was just under a year from the Appointed Day. The executive councils, which were to handle general medical and dental practice, pharmacy, and the supplementary ophthalmic services, were a modification of the old insurance committees, but even they required a lot of preparation. The county and county borough health committees, with their experienced medical officers of health, had lost direct hospital responsibilities but acquired wider functions in community support services. We were fortunate indeed not to have attempted to establish unitary health authorities, but rather the tripartite system that did ensure that all components of the NHS were properly supported. On 5 July 1948 everything *did* work.

Uneasy negotiations with doctors

There had been a very uneasy period of negotiation with the medical profession despite the Spens Committees on remuneration which had recommended increases for GPs. Even weeks before 5 July, there was still disagreement about GPs' pay and, in fact, an unfair settlement was forced through. But general practice was (and still is) the main component of health care in Britain. For the first time, all women and children had access to any necessary care and general medical practice carried that load. Because of the shortfall in remuneration, there was little opportunity for recruitment. There was, naturally, major disagreement between GPs and government and until the unfairness of the adjustment for inflation had been corrected, after Judge Danckwert's inquiry four years later, much needed changes did not occur. Oddly enough, that was to be helpful later, because the large additional sum awarded to GPs could be used, first, to secure a better system of distribution not solely based on capitation and, second, to provide financial inducements for group practice.

I think that it has too often been forgotten that the profession not only negotiated these changes willingly, but also volunteered a substantial sum annually from the pool of GPs' earnings to provide interest-free loans for group practices to improve their premises. A Royal Commission seven years later was to point out that this money should have come from the government, not from doctors' own pockets. This settlement led to immediate improvements in other ways, promoting moderate sized lists as well as group practice, but it still had serious defects which had to be corrected with the Family Doctors' Charter a dozen years later. The next step forward occurred with the association of health visitors and home nurses when this group of health professionals started working with group practices, a pattern then called attachment. Winchester and Oxford were the pioneers in a system which has emerged as the primary care of today. The idea was that of individuals locally, such as Ronald Gibson and John Warin, but by the mid 1960s it was widely accepted.

The College of General Practitioners founded in those early days was to become one of the most important influences on the NHS and the evolution of medicine in Britain. It put the continued learning which is essential to the profession at the forefront of its work and funded it where government did not.

Dentistry and optometry, like general practice, were suddenly available without impediment to many who had formerly been unable to afford them. The demand far exceeded the supply and the cost rose excessively and had to be adjusted. It took some three years for the supply of spectacles to catch up with demand. The supply of hearing aids was a new service using a design from the Medical Research Council and it took the hospital service years to reduce delays.

Local authority community services undervalued

The community services provided by local health authorities have too often been undervalued. Environmental hygiene and public provision of housing for the needy were a local responsibility and the old style of school health and maternity and child welfare still had its useful purpose, even though family doctor services were now free. But the broader basis of community support, including home nursing and home help, was important, especially with the increasing number of old people. Nearly two fifths of births still took place at home and this required an organised midwifery service, too.

Immunisation against diphtheria had been widespread from 1941 and new vaccines became available for other infections so that communicable disease ceased to be the major problem. It was the reduction in the load of infections, especially tuberculosis, which largely funded the real progress made in hospital services in the NHS's first dozen years.

The identification of smoking as the largest avoidable cause of premature death should have led to much stronger action against its commercial promotion than has been achieved even now, more than 40 years later. This was almost the first identification of the need for preventive action against non-infective disease needing central rather than local action. The social causes of wide class differences in mortality were to be clarified later by the Black report (see Chapter 3). Again, effective action has not been taken and no government has yet faced up to this. Commercial promotion of smoking was permitted despite the emphatic presentation of objections to it, notably by the Royal College of Physicians of London in its 1962 report and by its brainchild ASH since. I think that this failure may have cost us many tens of thousands of premature deaths and millions of years of productive life, a sorry chapter in Britain's health care.

Maternity services were changing and we had to take the opportunity to reduce both maternal and neonatal mortality. The triennial reports of the Confidential Enquiry into Maternal Deaths from 1952 and the succession of inquiries into neonatal mortality all helped to accentuate the trend towards hospital deliveries but also emphasised the need for better antenatal care. The Maternity Advisory Committee of the Central Health Services Council (CHSC) produced one of the earliest attempts at guidance in the clinical field with its report *Antenatal Care in Relation to Toxaemia of Pregnancy* and a later note on haemolytic disease of the newborn helped to improve practice. But the great need was for better joint working of midwives and doctors in and out of hospital, a need still not fully met. Even more important was to improve human relations in midwifery on which the advisory committee produced a later report. Real progress was slowly made, though there is yet more to do.

In a related field, *The Welfare of Children in Hospital* was another CHSC report which helped greatly to improve hospital care for children both here and abroad. It seems strange to recall now that some consultants even in the 1960s still insisted that children in hospital should not be visited, a fact which led to the sharpest admonition the Standing Medical Advisory Committee ever issued.

Hospital services required greatest changes

Hospital services required the greatest changes in the new NHS. I visited many buildings in the run-up to the Appointed Day and most were out of date, inadequately equipped, and often unsatisfactorily staffed. Yet the capital available in the first 12 years permitted only the most urgent additions of such facilities as operating theatres, laboratories, radiology departments, and outpatient services. The nationwide shortage of materials as well as of money meant that priority had to be given to housing, schools, and industry after the war. In a way, that prevented a rush to build on old, no longer suitable hospital plans but it also focused attention on the more important development of improved staffing. Capital for major new building became available in the 1960s and, fortunately, Enoch Powell, then Minister of Health, brought together regional schemes as a national plan. That meant that resources were used where needs were greatest and the concept of the district general hospital was central to it.

Though what was done was insufficient, at least the effort was directed to the right places. I recall how relatively easy it was to combine local hospitals

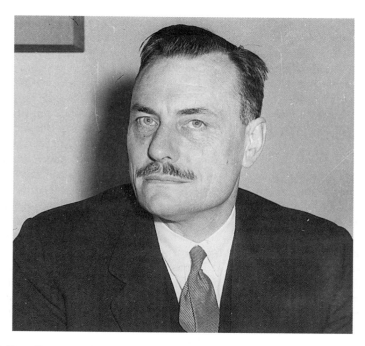

Enoch Powell was appointed Conservative Minister of Health in July 1960. In 1962 he unveiled the Goverment's *Hospital Plan for England and Wales,* an £800 million investment programme for a network of district general hospitals. Scotalnd had a similar plan. Reproduced with permission from Getty Images.

18

for better nurse training and the profession was responsive to this. By contrast, medical staffing outside the main centres required far more radical change and was harder to achieve. The NHS completed the separation of general and specialist practice and a strict (sometimes too strict, I thought) process of grading took place through regional professional committees. That left a measure of discontent among doctors that stumbled on for a decade, but it also opened the way for regionally planned recruitment and for the development of new specialties as required. By the time of the first radical administrative changes of the 1970s, a region/district pattern of specialist staffing was firmly established.

The number of consultants roughly doubled in the first 25 years, but the increase was not in the long established specialties of general medicine and surgery. The greatest total growth occurred in such specialties as anaesthesiology, psychiatry, pathology and, proportionately, in newer, smaller specialties such as radiotherapy, thoracic surgery, and cardiology. The most remarkable change occurred in the care of the elderly, where the new specialty of geriatrics and, later, psychogeriatrics showed how much could be done for those once labelled and virtually abandoned as the "chronic sick".

The change in psychiatry occurred in the same period because new psychotropic drugs and a quickly developing change in the professional attitudes of doctors, nurses, and social workers moved the emphasis from segregation to early active treatment and support in the community. The number of patients admitted in a year increased but the number in hospital at any one time was reduced by more than a half.

Inequalities in funding

Inequalities in funding were reduced only slowly, except for Scotland and Northern Ireland, both of which progressively gained substantial advantage. Much depended on the initiative of regional boards. But the discipline of the review of outcome, owed so largely to Professor Archie Cochrane, developed only gradually.

The process of change in hospital staffing brought a full range of specialist care to all. Within a region, the collaborative system meant that the most highly specialist service was as available to someone living in, say, a Cornish village, as it was to the patient's counterpart in Bristol, with NHS ambulances available if needed. But the system had defects, which arose as much from professional custom as from the structure. Hospital medical staff grew rapidly but in an unbalanced way. Delegation of work to junior staff may be possible but is not justified in my view if this simply increases their numbers and delays the advancement of their share in responsibility. It is even more important now that young minds should be introduced to control as soon as they are ready for it, than it was 45 years ago. In an odd way, the delaying influence of senior medical staff aided the central wish to reduce the rate of cost increase. A succession of expert committees reviewed hospital staffing until in 1969, Richard Crossman, Secretary of State for Social Services, accepted an increase of 500 consultants a year and a reduction in the number in lower grades. Sadly, the profession obstructed and reduced that change and the consequences are still with us.

Health professionals prefer collaboration to competition

- I could select many more examples than I have given of initiatives that advanced the NHS – or even examples of conflict or obstruction.
- Yet my impression after working with the health professions over 30 years of planning and development is of medical, nursing and other professional goodwill.
- The NHS does matter to nurses, doctors, dentists, pharmacists, and others working with patients in it.
- Health professionals seek to do their own work better, but they collaborate with each other rather than compete: they do not see themselves as selling items of care but as contributing to a whole – not to make it perfect but to do the best we can.

Scientific progress in medicine made increased specialisation and continuing education for doctors essential and it placed a special burden on general practice, which was and remains the guiding agent to secure the right specialist resource for the patients. At the end of 1961 a conference sponsored by the Nuffield Trust on medical postgraduate education led to an immediate response from the profession to establish postgraduate centres in every hospital group. Initially this was at doctors' own expense, but from two years later the NHS funded support. We all now accept the need for all doctors to receive continuing education, but that particular spontaneous effort was one of the most heartening examples of the central ethos of medicine. The agreement on the Family Doctors' Charter, which we owe to the skilful negotiations led by Kenneth Robinson for the government and James Cameron for GPs, was the only comparable episode.

3: Socioeconomic deprivation and the NHS: a complex relationship

Sir Douglas Black

I use the lengthy periphrasis "socioeconomic deprivation" instead of "poverty" not from any love of portentous terminology and still less from any wish to be "politically correct". I do so rather to emphasise the multifaceted nature of the disadvantages which beset those who, from no fault of their own, find themselves at the lower end of the social scale. They are not merely "poor" (the economic element) but are condemned to live in squalor, even sometimes without a home. They have no easy access to educational and cultural opportunities, nor indeed the leisure to enjoy them. They are also open to the contagion of unhealthy lifestyles, often promoted by unscrupulous advertising.

Unsurprisingly, such conditions fix a great gulf between their health experience and that description of health put forward by the World Health Organisation in the idealistic aftermath of the Second World War: "A state of complete physical, mental and social well-being, and not merely the absence of disease or infirmity".

If the picture which I have given of deprivation is in any way correct, practical consequences flow from it. The ill health associated with poverty has social roots and is therefore not susceptible to any "quick fix" by a health service which (in my view, quite correctly) has its major focus on illnesses and disabilities which are overt and in many cases can be cured or relieved. The relief of "minute particulars" is a legitimate task for any doctor. It will not in itself, however, ensure the "general good", which must be the concern of public health medicine. Full attainment of the general good cannot come from any type of medicine but only from the kind of "good society" called for by the influential economist J. K. Galbraith and others.

Even though the contribution of medicine to improving the health of the poor cannot be total, that does not make it negligible. In this chapter I assess the contribution of the NHS to that end. To do so, I shall try to give

21

a picture of health care at three periods: before the NHS was founded; in the years after it had become established; and as things are now. For the first two of these, I can draw on my direct experience as a clinician, but for the third I am a "non-participant" observer, except of course as a patient.

Before the Appointed Day

Qualifying in 1936, I worked mainly in hospital posts but was encouraged by my salary level to gain some experience of general practice as a locum, something which I have never regretted. The same would apply to my four years in the Royal Army Medical Corps. Furthermore, as the son of a minister with no independent means, I was spared the rigours of private schooling. Instead, I had an early opportunity of knowing schoolmates who were poorly clothed and nourished, one of whom died of rheumatic carditis before reaching his teens. And that was in a small town in which the jute mills were still giving employment, in contrast to areas of heavy manufacture where unemployment was severe. In my medical course, the cloistered privilege of St Andrews was followed by three years in Dundee, where poverty and its medical consequences were overt in the streets, in the wards of the Royal Infirmary, and in the homes which we entered in the pursuit of obstetric skills (fortunately accompanied by a midwife). Unemployment and, to an extent, poverty were soon to be palliated by the manpower needs of total war and these pseudo-benefits lasted into the early years of peace.

My direct experience of general practice, being limited to the prewar years, was not extensive. The patterns of provision, however, were plain to see. Those who could afford it (and some who could not) paid fees. The 1911 National Insurance Act provided primary care for about a sixth of male employees, those earning less than £160 per annum; for this privilege the employee paid four old pence a week, the balance of Lloyd George's "ninepence for fourpence" being provided by the employer (3d) and the state (2d). The scheme did not include women, children, retired workers, the self-employed or the unemployed; nor did it provide hospital treatment. For all the excluded categories, a family doctor was entitled to charge a fee, though in the face of real poverty many did not.

Cottage hospitals provided inpatient facilities in many smaller communities, as an extension of primary care, a site for minor surgery, and a place where a visiting surgeon could operate. In the cities, hospital care was provided in voluntary hospitals, municipal hospitals, and nursing homes. The voluntary hospitals were associated with medical schools and had an "honorary" senior staff, dependent on their private practice. They were financed by endowment, by voluntary contributions, by subscription schemes of relatively small individual payments, and by "flag days" and the like. Though prestigious national hospitals had accumulated substantial private funds, the general financing of voluntary hospitals had become precarious. A respite came early in the war, with state support of the Emergency Medical Service, which to an extent foreshadowed the NHS hospital service. Again, in the cities municipal hospitals funded by the local authorities provided services and were likewise to be incorporated in the future NHS.

This division was to provoke an important dispute between two heavyweight Labour ministers, Nye Bevan, Minister of Health, who favoured a national service, and Home Secretary Herbert Morrison, who wanted an extension of local authority provision. The battle was won by Bevan but the war against a fragmented health service has not been conclusively won. Nursing homes provided hospital care in a private sector which was very substantial, since specialists were dependent on it for a livelihood. Specialists and nursing homes varied in quality but the scope of medical care was much less, with fewer and probably "less specialised" specialists needed or available than is now the case. The need for surgery was more apparent than the need for medical specialism; in consequence, there were fewer specialist physicians than there were surgeons.

Paradoxically, this somewhat ramshackle system of health care did not specifically disadvantage the very poor, as regards access. In an emergency, they could be admitted to a voluntary or municipal hospital, at least in the cities. But of course, that still left them with the burdens of chronic illness and disability, to which they were differentially liable. The real victims of the health care system were the middle classes, who had to bear the cost of their own care. Their discontent must have been one of the political springs of the NHS.

Development of a national service

The birth pangs of the NHS have often been described, both by those at centre stage, such as Pater and Grey-Turner, and by retrospective analysts, for example, Klein and Timmins. My concern here is with a later stage of the NHS, in the 1960s, when the sharp conflicts had died away, the service had won the confidence of patients and staff, and a Tory health minister, Iain Macleod, had felt able to say in 1958, "The National Health Service, with the exception of recurring spasms about charges, is out of party politics". By that time, widespread approval for a nationwide service, funded to a large extent from general taxation, had replaced earlier misgivings as it became manifest that health care, previously limited to a minority of the people, had now become comprehensively available. Every citizen was entitled to the care of a family doctor and could be referred for specialist care at his discretion, with at first no direct charge to the patient for any of the services. Later on, prescription charges and other fees were introduced, as it became apparent that the Beveridge expectation, that costs would diminish once a backlog of untreated but treatable illness had been disposed of, was not to be fulfilled. Indeed, the increased scope for effective medical and surgical intervention would call for greater funding.

In the early years of the service, there was an emphasis on development of hospitals, including both greater sophistication in existing hospitals and the establishment of district hospitals throughout the land. Patients were even at one time inclined to dismiss what could be achieved in primary care and to make demands for inappropriate specialist care. This led to low morale among family doctors, who rightly perceived themselves as undervalued. Happily, the Family Doctors' Charter negotiated in 1966 between Jim Cameron, the BMA's GP leader, and Labour's health minister, Kenneth Robinson, secured decent terms and conditions of service. The earlier founding of the Royal College of General Practitioners had brought an added stimulus to training and morale.

In 1977, as the 30th anniversary of the NHS approached, David Ennals set up a working party to study "inequalities in health between the social classes". Perhaps he did this in the hope that the well recognised disadvantage to health associated with poverty might have been lessened by the greater availability of medical care brought about by the NHS. [*The author chaired that working party. Ed.*] Disappointingly, the gap was not only greater than had been supposed, but had actually widened since 1948. On the other hand, the health of all groups had improved, most notably in infancy. These superficially discordant findings stimulated a wealth of speculation and clearly many factors are involved. To suggest two general factors: first, in tackling ill health due largely to social causes, remedial care is only a palliative, important though that may be for the individual; second, the benefits available from the NHS may have been more efficiently taken up by the middle classes than by the very poor. This is particularly so for health education and it is notable that the incidence of coronary heart disease has fallen much more in non-manual workers than in manual workers, especially among the unskilled.

Farewell, consensus

In the 17th century William Harvey, endowing his Oration (given annually at the Royal College of Physicians of London), maintained the value of consensus, claiming that given "concord", small beginning could become great, but that with "discord", even great things would fall apart. Perhaps it is just as well that I cannot here consider the general aspect of the 1991 "reforms" of the health service. It is relevant, however, to draw attention to their multiple divisiveness – "purchaser" has been set against "provider", when they should be united in a common purpose. The balance between family doctors and hospital doctors has been moved from discussion to economic power.

Family doctors are themselves divided over fundholding. Transfer of patients to the most appropriate place or form of care, previously made by informal arrangement, is now constrained by the exigencies of contracts, which serve no purpose but that of the internal pseudo-market. And, of course, financial competition between rival trusts is a recipe for general disharmony in what should be an integrated hospital system. Common sense suggests that allocating limited resources effectively in such a complex and socially sensitive service as health care needs co-ordination, not competition.

The future

I believe that:
- though the 1990s market changes distract attention and withdraw resources from the main purpose of the NHS, they are not differentially harmful to the very poor;
- paradoxically, the shift of emphasis from specialist to primary care may bring greater awareness of the health disadvantages of poverty, for family doctors are more integrated into their community than a specialist working in what may be a distant hospital;
- to translate awareness of the disadvantages into actual benefit will require from society a planned attack on poverty itself;
- it will require from doctors and other health workers a deliberate reversal of Tudor Hart's "inverse care law", which suggests that those most in need of care receive the least;
- the 1995 report on *Variations in Health* from the Department of Health engenders some optimism because it showed both concern for the problem of poverty and poor health and recognition that it calls for a widely based strategy, if progress is to be made, as of course it should be;
- A further reason for guarded optimisim is that the Labour Government is now committed to a broad strategy to combat health inequalities;
- The appointment in May 1997 of a Minister for Public Health, and the setting up of a group chaired by Sir Donald Acheson suggests that the health consequences of social deprivation are being taken seriously. That does not make the problems easier or less complex; but the emergence of a will to solve them is new and encouraging.

4: Politics and the NHS

Lord Owen

Britain's National Health Service has over its first 50 years been subjected to innumerable reorganisations and financial and administrative reviews. Despite or because of that and against all predictions its essential framework has remained intact. Today central government still provides a nationwide service, financed out of general taxation with general practitioners as independent contractors and hospital consultants permitted to conduct private practice in addition to their NHS practice.

Making the people healthier did not, as was hoped, reduce the pressure on the NHS. Instead, health demand increased and costs rose. A longstanding controversy between the politicians and the medical profession has been whether the NHS was providing a comprehensive service. Public expenditure on health care has substantially increased and many services have expanded but still some parts of the health service have had to be restricted. For example, the dental service no longer even pretends to offer comprehensive cover.

The NHS has survived as it is because of political compromises, often hard fought on ideological grounds within government as well as outside with the health professions – both of which I can personally testify to. It is not possible to understand the NHS today without reflecting on what might have been if three ideological clashes involving six of the more colourful of our politicians had turned out differently. These clashes were between Aneurin Bevan and Herbert Morrison on the nationalisation of the hospitals; between Barbara Castle and Harold Wilson on the phasing out of pay beds; and between Margaret Thatcher and Nigel Lawson on tax concessions for private medicine.

Looking back from the end of the 20th century, it is easy to assume that it was inevitable that a health service under the Attlee government would come under central government control and be answerable for all its activity to the Westminster Parliament. In fact, Herbert Morrison as Lord President of the Council, Leader of the House and, unofficially, deputy Prime Minister assumed that the new NHS would come under local government. He argued that nationalisation of all hospitals, as proposed by Aneurin

Bevan, deprived local government of one of its major functions. This was the big change from the plan hammered out in the wartime Coalition Government and published in the 1944 White Paper.

Aneurin Bevan argued successfully that it was unsound to leave local government with a service largely financed by the Exchequer. Bevan's biographer, Michael Foot, describes this as his biggest battle and "the most crucial in the whole fight for the Health Service". The London County Council (LCC) was, in 1945, the largest hospital authority in the country and the largest public health authority in the world. Morrison, who had been a skilful leader of the LCC, was not a man to be easily overturned. "He lived politics, ate politics, dreamt politics . . . he had a finger in every pie". The fact that Bevan beat him in Cabinet is a sign of how formidable was Bevan's mastery of his brief and his ministry within months of taking office. It is also why Bevan deserves the accolade of being the creator of the NHS.

Conflict between politicians and doctors inevitable

Conflicts between politicians and the medical profession are inevitable and did not start with the creation of the NHS. Lloyd George as Chancellor of the Exchequer in June 1911, in a speech in Birmingham Town Hall, revealed the rawness of his relationship with the doctors. "I do not think there has been anything like it since the days when Daniel went into the lions' den . . . but I can assure you they treated me with the same civility as the lions treated my illustrious predecessor . . . except these lions knew their anatomy".

When financial times are difficult, doctors have a habit of recycling the old cry that politics should be kept out of the health service, to which a wise old parliamentarian is reported to have retorted that it would be easier to keep patients out of the health service.

For the run-up to the launch of the NHS, Aneurin Bevan faced a powerful BMA led by Guy Dain, its Chairman, and the "radio doctor" Charles Hill, its Secretary. The BMA held a plebiscite in December 1946 when 54% of the profession voted against co-operating on framing the regulations for the new service. Dain, in speeches, referred to Bevan as the "Medical Service Dictator" and Hill declaimed against a choice between "Bevan or Belsen". My own GP father was one of the 46% who voted in favour of discussion and later greeted the start of the NHS, on 5 July 1948, as a day of freedom when he never needed again to ask a patient to pay for his services.

Bevan's famous explanation for the BMA's eventual acceptance of the NHS related to the consultants: "I stuffed their mouths with gold". But Bevan never downplayed the intensity of the whole profession's passionate belief that their clinical freedom was bound up in the right to private practice, a view held even by those doctors who never wished to charge any patient and were ready to practise whole time within the NHS. Bevan was also pragmatic in 1949 about introducing prescription charges, telling audiences, "I shudder to think of the ceaseless cascade of medicine which is pouring down British throats at the present time", a comment which made his later resignation over NHS charges look less than principled. The Labour left, however, never forgave the medical profession for supposedly wringing the concession of the right to practise private medicine within the NHS out of their hero, Nye.

Angry doctors

Twice Labour, voted back into government, faced an angry medical profession: in 1964, the general practitioners and in 1974, the hospital consultants. On both occasions the frustrations had built up under Conservative governments. In 1964 GPs were threatening to withdraw from the NHS. A decade later, on 11 June 1974, the BMA called on consultants to resign unless their pay review body came up with large increases and the government introduced a contract based on "fee for service" remuneration. Consultants wanted the BMA to set up its own employment agency to hire their services back to the NHS. The nurses were also in a rather more justified ferment about their miserable pay.

Suddenly, the problems of a highly centralised health service exploded in the press and Parliament. Granny, "Ma" or "Mrs" Brookstone, depending on which paper one read, was leading a strike of NUPE members in the NHS against the use of the private wing on the 15th floor of Charing Cross Hospital. The local health authority compromised with their shop stewards, but the BMA decided to take up the issue directly with the Secretary of State, Barbara Castle, and make it an issue of principle – provoked in part by the *Daily Mail* headline, "Give in . . . or we will starve the patients out". Suddenly, for the hospital consultants pay and private practice were fused into one. I, as Minister of Health, chairing a working party on the consultants' contract, was in the centre of a maelstrom. The Labour Party's manifesto commitment to "phase out private practice from the hospital service" was itself a hard-won concession from those on the Labour left, who wanted a statutory ban. It was seen by the doctors as the thin end of the wedge. Barbara Castle retained the support of the Labour and Liberal parties in Parliament and tried to reassure the consultants that she was not trying to reverse Aneurin Bevan's compromise and impose a whole-time salaried service by the backdoor, (but merely geographically separating private from public beds). Too many in the profession, however, were not prepared to believe her. As the junior doctors were also threatening to strike over long working hours, I remember once saying to her "Even Nye with an overall majority close to 150 did not have the consultants, GPs and junior doctors against him. We have to compromise".

Lord Goodman, Harold Wilson's solicitor, was advising the BMA. Barbara Castle was under no illusion that if she did not compromise with Arnold Goodman, Harold Wilson, on this issue the pragmatist, would undercut her in Cabinet and force a settlement, for Wilson could sense the public mood was turning.

Eventually a compromise was negotiated in which pay beds were to be

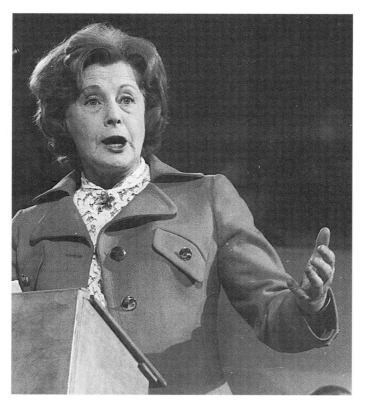

Barbara Castle (later Baroness Castle). Secretary of State for Social Services from 1974 to 1976 during Harold Wilson's second term as Labour Prime Minister, she clashed with hospital doctors over the Government's plans to remove private beds from NHS hospitals. Lord Owen, Minister of Health at the time, chaired a joint working party with the medical profession to resolve the conflict. The mix of state and private sector medicine had originally been agreed by Aneurin Bevan to persuade hospital doctors to enter the NHS in 1948. Reproduced with permission from Getty Images.

phased out slowly but under legislative safeguards by an independent Health Service Board, ensuring that there had to be alternative private facilities available. The consultants got more money and dropped their demand for item of service payments. The Conservative government elected in 1979 abolished the Board, retained pay beds and allowed whole-time consultants to do some private practice.

It was a welcome change that New Labour in 1997 came into government with no commitment to challenge the role of private medicine in the pattern of British health care. It was easier for New Labour to change its approach in the 1990s because of what happened in 1988 when Margaret Thatcher was Prime Minister.

Thatcher and Lawson at odds over tax concessions on private care

Margaret Thatcher had an equal, though opposite, ideological commitment to private medicine as had Barbara Castle. She was repulsed by her own Chancellor of the Exchequer, Nigel Lawson. It had been obvious for some time that Margaret Thatcher was biding her time until after the 1987 election before launching a fundamental challenge to the NHS. She knew the NHS was popular and that only a series of steps towards financing it through private insurance would be acceptable even to her own party. She had, for similar reasons, rejected a wide extension of charging NHS patients.

What she put to the small five-member ministerial group under her chairmanship set up on 28 January 1988 to review the NHS was to make all subscriptions to private health insurance schemes tax deductible and to cease to tax as a benefit in kind the provision of private health care to employees under a company scheme. Lawson vigorously opposed this and in a note to the committee, succinctly and brutally put the contrary view from a Conservative standpoint, the first time the issue had been fully examined by a Conservative government since 1945. "If we simply boost demand, for example, by tax concessions to the private sector, without improving supply, the result would be not so much a growth in private health care, but higher prices". He warned, "The key is the supply side, as we have recognised in most other areas of policy. Moreover, of course, increasing demand in the private sector pushes up prices and therefore pay. That would inevitably spread across all staff costs in the NHS, and we would end up getting less value for money". Lawson reluctantly offered a facesaver to Mrs Thatcher of tax relief for contributions from old age pensioners. If this was the greatest inroad into the structure of the NHS that the Conservative's greatest ideologue could achieve, it was not hard for New Labour to rebuff its left wing supporters.

Predicated health tax should be the future

- A modified, less bureaucratic purchaser/provider system will not be sufficient to last far into the 21st century.
- Public opinion consistently shows that people are prepared to support an earmarked and quite specific NHS tax and could accept this increasing, while income tax was held steady or declined.
- Earmarking or predicating tax for a specific purpose is, as always, opposed by the Treasury; nevertheless, I hope to see such a tax introduced.
- Then our NHS will provide higher standards of care for everyone.

Much will depend on whether the concept of an internal market survives well into the 21st century. These reforms did not start with the Conservatives but were advocated first by Alain Enthoven, an American, who had served as a Democrat in the US Defence Department under Robert MacNamara and who later became professor at the Stanford School of Business. His concept was then championed by the Social Democratic Party in 1984 against a wall of official scepticism. So much so that the Conservative government rushed out criticism from the Health Service Management Board in 1986, before the 1987 election, rebuffing the internal market. Yet these same reforms then became the centrepiece of the Conservative government's health review in November 1988. The reforms drew a clear distinction between the financing and the purchase of health care and it is this which provides an internal market, where NHS costs become transparent. It is, however, not privatisation.

New Labour are dropping the term "market" but keeping the internal purchaser/provider separation in the NHS, adjusting bureaucratic proce-dures in the light of experience. The government has also stopped tax relief for private health care. In this way the NHS will enter the 21st century retaining the essential framework laid down in 1945. Different governments will argue about the best way of controlling spiralling health costs while ensuring that even individuals with a poor health record have open access.

5: The NHS and the national health

George Davey Smith

The National Health Service in 1948 was an inevitable consequence of the period which preceded it. Memories of the depression, coupled with experience of the social integration which accompanies mobilisation for war, encouraged the popular perception of health care as a right, not a privilege. Advocates of a publicly funded comprehensive health service invoked the poor health of those in poverty and inequalities in health between social groups as indicators of the need for an integrated care system. The extent to which the working class wanted adequate health care was shown by people's willingness to contribute from low wages to friendly society and sick club health insurance schemes, as well as in active campaigning and agitation for a better health service. Behind this activity lay the perception that medical services improved health and life expectancy. In an avowedly activist book in 1937, the socialist historians G.D.H. and M.I. Cole wrote:

> Doctoring of a fairly competent sort is now within the reach of a far larger proportion of the people than it used to be; and some part of the fall in the death rate and of the general improvement of health over the past two decades is attributable to this cause.

From a different perspective, H.M. Vernon, former investigator for the Industrial Health Research Board, considered that bad social conditions adversely influenced health, but he argued that:

> Something can be done to reduce the harmful influence by introducing various remedial measures. One of the most important of such measures is the provision of a thoroughly efficient medical service, by means of which everyone, however poor, can obtain the best advice and treatment.

While life expectancy had increased and health had improved since the turn of the century, the Coles and Vernon considered Britain to have worse health than many comparable countries. Gross inequalities in wealth were thought to lead to both large inequalities in health and a nation with poor overall health. While health inequalities and poor health in general needed to be dealt with at the broad societal level, improved health services and more equal access to these services were also important.

Mortality rates in Britain started their long decline in the 1860s, beginning in the youngest post-infant age group and then, in cohort fashion, extending into the older age groups. The decline of infant mortality awaited the arrival of the post-1860 cohorts of women into the childbearing age group. By the second decade of the 20th century death rates were declining at all ages. During the depression of the 1930s infant mortality continued to fall, though some economically deprived areas were exceptions to this rule. As infant mortality was seen to be highly responsive to social conditions, its continued decline was somewhat unexpected. Life expectancy for men over 40 and women over 50, however, showed small falls between 1921 and 1940 and evidence of poor nutritional status among children was widespread. The health of the unemployed and of manual workers was an issue of considerable concern. To compound this, the health care available to most of the population, often paid for from hard earned and inadequate salaries, was self-evidently highly unsatisfactory.

NHS expected to improve health

Against this background, the introduction of a National Health Service was expected to produce both improved health and a more equitable society. In the words of (then) Major Jerry Morris:

> A single tax for health, granting in return and without further ado the right to all health services, would be a giant stride towards simpler living and a healthier and better Britain. The president of the Society of Medical Officers of Health described the National Health Service Act as "the greatest thing that had ever been done in social medicine in any age or country".

There is some irony, then, in the fact that practitioners of social medicine came to view health services as being of little importance to the health of populations. The "liberal retreat", as J.J. Hart described it, is most closely associated with the work of Thomas McKeown, whose central claim was that long term declines in mortality in Britain were primarily the outcome of improved nutrition and hygiene. The contribution of clinical medicine was viewed as minor, even after the introduction of antibiotics in 1972. Archie Cochrane, in a monograph for the Nuffield Provincial Hospitals Trust, elegantly identified the degree to which medical therapeutics was an act of faith rather than science. He strongly advocated the role of randomised trials in identifying which components of health care did more harm than good. Cochrane then discussed various indicators of health service activity, including the number of doctors, nurses and hospital beds per unit population size and the percentage of gross national product spent on health. He found infant mortality to be positively related to density of doctors, as was adult mortality up to middle age. Of 70 possible associations between indicators of health service activity and mortality outcomes, 46 were in the direction of greater activity indicating worse mortality: none of the 24 associations in the other direction was statistically significant.

Nutrition, environment, and behaviour determine health

The best known of the academic critiques of the importance of medical care, that of Tom McKeown in 1976, was primarily concerned with historical trends in mortality in Britain. It could be accepted as an accurate assessment of what had happened in the past but not necessarily of relevance to the present experience of mortality transitions. McKeown certainly intended the extrapolation to be made, however, claiming that:

> In order of importance the determinations of health were nutritional, environ-
> mental and behavioural in the past, and will probably be behavioural,
> environmental and nutritional in the future, at least in developed countries.

The critiques of the effects of medical care, advances from various perspectives by other commentators, elicited many responses. For example, in 1991 S.J. Kunitz denied that it had ever been considered that medical care had a serious influence on health. This is a difficult position to maintain if we assess all relevant professional and lay comments. Indeed, initial experiences of antimicrobial agents led doctors to believe, not surprisingly perhaps, that they were seriously influencing mortality. A second reaction was to suggest that it is not possible to develop sensible indicators of the effects of medical care on health. This was coupled with the suggestion that some aspects of medical care – reassurance and the general "Samaritan role" of medicine – could not be quantified and levels of general health and functioning, as opposed to mortality rates, could not be tracked over time. A third approach, advocated by J.M. Winter in 1982, has been to claim that interventions which do not require a medical qualification to implement – such as dietary or hygiene advice – should be considered medical interventions when they have come from the health sector. The contribution of formal medicine both to the knowledge base and to the legitimisation of the message is, in this view, of importance.

A more radical response to the "McKeown hypothesis" has been simply to reject its central premise. S. Szreter in 1958 emphasised the importance of directed social intervention, through wide ranging public health and preventive measures, including municipal sanitation, housing improvement, health education, and food hygiene (including treatment of milk), as opposed to the unmotivated effects of abstract economic improvement. The medical input into these activities at all levels was substantial and therefore claims for the effectiveness of medicine in its broadest, and particularly public health, formulation are being made. In a broader defence of medical care, Johansson suggested that the impact of the personal physician on health was relevant. He saw the influence of clinical practice on population health as initially small, because only elite groups received useful care. Johansson put forward various aspects of the clinical encounter which could benefit health, suggesting that as these became available more widely and as medical knowledge and techniques advanced, influences on the overall health of population became apparent.

British mortality trends and effect of medical care

British mortality trends in the second half of the 20th century show continuing declines in mortality for men under 65 and women under 85; for older ages, declines only resumed in the 1970s. Infectious and parasitic diseases in all age groups and circulatory disease (mostly rheumatic heart disease) in children all showed accelerated falls in mortality immediately after the war. With the exception of 25–44 year-old men, the falls in mortality at younger ages have accelerated from the mid 1970s, with falling rates of circulatory and respiratory mortality contributing most to this. For people over 60, the falls in mortality among British men in the 1980s were among the most impressive seen in Europe. Morbidity trends are more difficult to measure, leaving unanswered the question as to the extent to which improved life expectancy comes at the expense of a longer period in ill health.

John Buckner, in 1995, estimated the extent to which medical care has influenced mortality trends. He used the most rigorous available data – from randomised trials, if possible – as the source of evidence on effectiveness. Grouping effective clinical preventive services (including screening for and treatment of detected hypertension; immunisation for diphtheria, polio and tetanus and screening for cervical cancer) and clinical therapies (including appendectomy; insulin for type I diabetes; treatment of kidney failure and ischaemic heart disease), he estimated that in the United States medical care had contributed about a fifth to the 30 years of increased life expectancy seen this century. While conceding that improvements in quality of life and reductions in morbidity have been more difficult to identify and evaluate, Buckner also claimed that medical care had made a meaningful contribution in this domain.

We must recognise several limitations of this exercise. Firstly, clinical trials are carried out on highly selected groups of patients and with careful monitoring of therapy. When implemented through routine health services, the outcomes may be much less favourable, as has been claimed for antihypertensive therapy. Secondly, adverse effects in medical treatments are not taken into account. These can be substantial and can result from unevaluated therapies being widely used. Examples are the 5500 deaths attributed to the inappropriate use of clofibrate in the US or the effect of the widespread use of antiarrhythmic therapy following myocardial infarction, a treatment which was later found to increase mortality. Peach and Charlton in 1986 pointed to more general adverse effects of medical care, including overmedication in particular.

Greater mortality falls among affluent groups

If medical care contributes to health, then a National Health Service, to the extent to which it leads to more equitable distribution of medical care, could have an important influence on population health. In England and Wales mortality amenable to medical care showed greater relative declines between 1931 and 1961 in the more affluent sections of society; between 1961 and 1981 the picture was less consistent. Jerry Morris and I have identified an overall pattern of greatly increasing relative and absolute mortality differentials between social groups since 1951. Furthermore, Payne and Saul have shown that for one potential intervention which can lower mortality – coronary revascularisation surgery – people living in more deprived areas have about half the rate of procedures of people in affluent areas, once the prevalence of angina is taken into account.

More children in poverty sow seeds of greater future inequalities

The Child Poverty Action Group warned, in 1977, that the recent social policies which have led to marked widening of inequalities in income and a dramatic increase in the percentage of children growing up in poverty may be sowing the seeds of even greater inequality in the future. If this occurs, the promise of the NHS will not be met.

While imprisoned for an editorial he wrote for the paper *Freedom* at the end of the war, Dr John Hewetson reflected on the future of the proposed national health service. He considered that the reforms on offer:

> . . . presuppose the continued existence of rich and poor. We can, therefore, say with conviction that they have not attempted to remove the root cause of ill-health - namely, poverty. These reforms will be as ineffective as those introduced since 1911.

With respect to continuing – and worsening – inequalities in wealth and health, Hewetson has been proved correct. Overall mortality, however, has improved substantially since the war and health services will have contributed in some part to this. Those groups which are showing the most dramatic declines in mortality, the 45–64 year-olds, were born or grew up during the war or the immediate postwar period and have benefited from the egalitarian policies, particularly with respect to nutrition, education, and health care, instituted at that time. The long term effects of these experiences on adult health will contribute to declining mortality.

6: From administration to management

Brian Edwards

It was Roy Griffiths, the Managing Director of Sainsbury's the grocers, who moved the NHS from administration to management in the early 1980s. The first Thatcher-led government had asked him to review the management of the NHS workforce in the wake of the industrial disputes in 1982. He and his team quickly concluded that the brave but flawed experiment in consensus management, launched in 1974, was not working in the tough and complex world of the NHS. As he vividly observed: "If Florence Nightingale were carrying her lamp through the corridors of the NHS today she would almost certainly be searching for the people in charge". Yet another NHS reorganisation had been spawned.

In a report marked by clarity and an economy of words, he called for every health authority and hospital to have a general manager, a streamlined managerial process with commercial style boards and a substantial devolution of decision making to unit level (usually a hospital or set of community services). A service that since 1948 had been administered rather than managed was about to undergo a revolution to a management culture.

Roy Griffiths was convinced that NHS staff were insufficiently valued and surprised that doctors did not contribute more to the management of the service. We can also trace back to this report the first serious managerial thinking about clinical audit and health outcomes, an overdue change in a traditionally provider driven service.

As a former NHS regional manager, I recall the fearsome survival process that managers had to negotiate to keep a senior post for any length of time. The regular cycle of reorganisation meant that we had to compete for whatever senior posts then became available. When the whole system changed, the manager had to compete with his peers on either a national or a regional basis. When the change was stimulated by local considerations (such as a merger), the local candidates usually fought it out head to head. Only the most resilient survived this process. It reinforced the mobility of talented managers, which undoubtedly enriched their experience. The downside was that it also separated us from senior doctors, who were not at all mobile and who had to keep adjusting to another new manager.

As the NHS absorbed the Griffiths organisational changes in 1983 the competition started at the regional level and cascaded down. The Department of Health was worried lest all the new management jobs went to existing administrators. Management needed to be seen to be different. New blood had to be recruited both from clinical disciplines and the private sector. An unofficial quota was set, the world and his dog were invited to apply, and the conclusions of local selection committees had to be approved by the tier above.

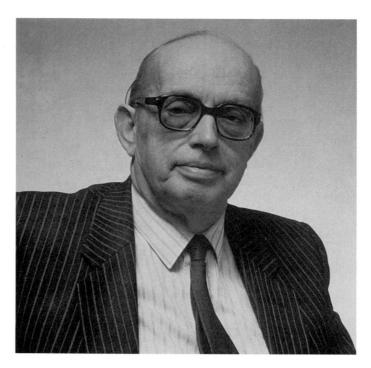

Sir Roy Griffiths. At the Conservative Government's request, Roy Griffiths, managing director of a supermarket chain, and three other businessmen reviewed how the NHS was managed. The recommendations in their brief report were quickly accepted by Norman Fowler, Secretary of State for Social Services, and the outcome was a revolution in the NHS's management structures and functions. Reproduced with permission from Sainsbury archives.

Old scores settled

Often local judgements were deemed unacceptable (some old scores were settled) and I remember some notable casualties among leading administrators. The first occupants of the regional general manager posts included people drawn from medical, nursing, accounting, and commercial backgrounds. The final analysis for the whole service showed that 60% of the jobs had gone to administrators and 11% to doctors and nurses, while 10% came from outside the NHS altogether. Quite a few appointees came from the Armed Forces but few survived for long.

In my case I had to compete for the regional post in Trent against a doctor with whom I had worked closely and for whom I had great respect – Professor James Scott. The interviews were held in Sheffield, with external assessors, and we both had to wait some weeks for a minister to approve the local recommendation, without either of us being told what it was. In the event, I was appointed and Jim, who remained Regional Medical Officer, and I worked closely together until he retired. Had I not been appointed I would have had to move and compete for one of the managerial jobs at district level. The new managerial role, while different, took the heart out of the job of the administrator at all levels. Like all general managers, I had to accept a short term contract of three years with no guarantee of continued employment in the NHS if it was not renewed. For this I received an increase of £3000 per annum.

Those of us appointed had a demanding but exciting time. As members of commercial style boards, we found an environment shorn of bureaucracy where action and results were the watchwords. Despite much talk about managerial culture and process, the system was not yet ready to embrace the notion of a full blown chief executive. He or she (there were a few women) was the leader of the team.

At a national level, the Secretary of State for Health and Social Services, Norman Fowler, chaired a new Supervisory Board and Victor Paige was headhunted from the recently privatised National Freight Company to become the first chairman of the NHS's National Management Board, another innovation. He had a refreshingly direct style but lasted only 17 months. Oddly, given the culture of management imposed on the NHS, the principles of general management had not extended into the Department of Health and he resigned in frustration. Len Peach, whom he had recruited as the first Director of Personnel, succeeded him. It took another six years for the national job to be filled by somebody with a NHS background: Duncan Nichol in 1989.

The attitude of the health professions to all of this was pretty negative, particularly when the Chief Nursing Officer in England did not get a seat on the National Board. Eventually, political pressure from within the service forced a change of heart. In the field, the negative attitudes faded as the pace of decision making did, indeed, improve.

Devolution process impeded

Everybody had applauded the policy of devolving decision making to unit level. In practice, however, the devolution process was impeded by officials at the higher tiers and by health authorities who wanted to retain power for themselves. Real devolution would have to wait for the radical innovation of NHS trusts in 1991.

The day to day agenda for the new general managers was occupied with building new teams and responding to a rash of efficiency studies undertaken by Sir Derek Rayner, Managing Director of Marks and Spencer. He reviewed nurses' homes, advertising, energy, and many other support services, a review hampered by another spate of industrial action. The cause was a mixture of pay and the government's policy of compulsory competitive tendering for support services. Trade unions were not alone in fighting this policy; many health authorities disliked it too. Ministers used strong arm tactics, however, and the policy was eventually forced on the NHS. Most contracts were awarded to in-house teams but with substantial financial savings and inevitable job losses.

In primary care, things went on much as usual, except for a noisy spat between ministers and doctors about the introduction of a limited list of prescribable NHS drugs. Ministers had been persuaded to re-establish independent family practitioner committees (FPCs) but this took years to push through Parliament. These committees got their own general managers in 1989 (with a few notable exceptions, they were a weak bunch) but in the 1990s drive for a slimmer bureaucracy, FPCs were amalgamated with health authorities . . . again.

In mental health, the large institutions were slowly closing as specialist community services expanded. Many a management board meeting was absorbed with the complicated business of selling off the extensive buildings and land.

In Trent, the managerial community turned its attention to the patient focused, quality agenda, developing a successful programme that ran under the name of Personal Service. It encouraged staff of all disciplines to see services through the eyes of the patient and empowered them to make local changes.

Power at the top

At the top of the service, the regular monthly meetings of regional general managers with civil servants were very powerful in shaping policy, as were the more political meetings between regional chairs and ministers. Both groups shared a full-time secretariat based in London.

These meetings had a great influence on shaping NHS activities but one of the most powerful national changes during this whole period was the introduction of the performance review process. My chairman and I presented ourselves at the Elephant and Castle NHS headquarters, to be asked by Norman Fowler the deceptively simple question: "What have you achieved with all the millions the government has invested in your region?". We struggled for a convincing answer but did a lot better the following year, when Kenneth Clarke was the minister asking the questions. We asked this question of all health authorities in the region on our return home. This was powerful stuff and gave real bite to the managerial process. Ministers, however, lost interest quite quickly (it was hard work and required them really to understand the special problems and issues in each region) but the system survived well into the next decade.

In Trent, we took the process very seriously indeed. The meetings were well prepared and thorough in their analysis of what had happened and what had been achieved in the previous year on each patch. Sir Michael Carlisle, Trent's chairman, and I shared the interrogation process. My objective on each occasion was to be sufficiently well briefed to be able to more than cope with the district manager and his team on the other side of the table. The meetings typically lasted three or four hours and attendance was compulsory for both chairs, general managers and their management teams. At the end of each meeting I did a full verbal summary, which included agreed tasks and targets for the following year. This summary was subsequently published, often to the discomfort of DHA chairs when it contained critical comments. For the most part, though, the public letters highlighted progress and success, of which there was a great deal. Services in Trent were expanding fast as money from the redistributive formula operated by the Resource Allocation Working Party (RAWP) continued to flow in.

RAWP narrowed regional disparities

This national formula allocated cash differentially between regions and when RAWP disappeared in 1987 it had successfully narrowed the investment gap between the south east of England and the rest of the country. Even in a gaining region like Trent, however, significant variation still persisted between health authorities. This was always the tension zone when we in our turn had to decide who would get what from the allocation Trent had received from London. The speed with which individual authorities moved towards notional equity was a matter for regions to determine unless the noise of local politics reached Westminster and ministers got involved. In Trent, we always set our face against actually reducing allocations for some in order to give to others, on the grounds that our high spenders were still below the national average. These authorities received only minimal growth and it left them living constantly on the margins of a financial crisis. Much energy was invested in RAWP arguments but in my view it was mainly misplaced, for the formula was always sensitive to "fine tuning" to ensure the answers it produced were sensible and politically correct.

Jim Scott and I as regional officers spent a deal of our time embroiled in the problems of disciplining hospital consultants, who were at this time employed by regional health authorities (unless they were in a teaching hospital). Neither of us was prepared to look away when incompetence or neglect was drawn to our attention, but all too often we found ourselves fighting a system designed to protect the poor performer. The system is only marginally better today.

The future

I foresee:
- an NHS free at the point of need and located primarily in the public sector being safe for the next decade, but with national investment continuing to be modest, arguments over rationing will become fiercer;
- the debate on clinical effectiveness and outcomes maturing into strong guidelines for effective and proper clinical practice;
- patients expecting an extended range of personal choice and more say in shaping the system itself;
- a highly professional primary care sector as vital to success but only with a rigorous programme of quality assurance;
- the hospital world becoming more integrated as specialisation increases;
- major clinical breakthroughs in those diseases where it is possible to develop integrated pathways of care that focus the skills of many professionals on individual patients;
- the pay of health service staff continuing to be a point of contention with government.

Building the network of district general hospitals (DGH) was well under way in most parts of the country by the mid 1980s and the process of funding them with topsliced money – funds centrally earmarked from a region's budget for spending on specific projects – was still in place. There were many royal openings, which were great social occasions as long as you avoided the enormously detailed preparation and the arguments about who would be on the receiving line. Even as these new hospitals opened, concern was mounting about the number of additional acute beds being built. Those who raised these worries were not popular. The concept of the comprehensive DGH was very strong and dominated all strategic thinking. Ten years on, the arguments continue.

The switch from administration to management was long and often traumatic. But the period was one of growth and development for the hospital world in particular. General management led to great improvements in the way the NHS was run. Strategic planning reached its high point but was creating the foundations for the financial crisis that lay ahead.

7: From singlehanded GP to team practice

Arnold Elliott

Brought up as a member of a middle class family in Belfast, I nevertheless realised how widespread was poverty in the province with unemployment the highest in the United Kingdom. Many women were shoddily dressed – the "shawlies" – children went about barefoot, and obvious signs of malnutrition, like rickets, were all too evident. As a medical student at Queen's University, I witnessed the diseases associated with poverty. Tuberculosis was rife, both as respiratory and skeletal infections. Affected patients filled many hospital wards. And from early on, I was conscious of the strong link between social factors and health.

After being demobbed from the Royal Army Medical Corps, I did a postservice registrarship at Lambeth Hospital. A large, grim London County Council hospital, which had previously been a Poor Law institution, it contained many hundreds of patients but few doctors to look after them. For me, however, this meant excellent clinical experience. The hospital was in an area of deprivation and we treated many down and outs from nearby Rowton House, a dosshouse for the homeless.

Together with many young people who had survived the war, I saw it as medically imperative to serve the community. I resolved to go into general practice and welcomed the introduction of the NHS. In particular, I was pleased to be able to treat patients irrespective of their ability to pay. Entering a singlehanded general practice in Ilford, Essex (now part of the London Borough of Redbridge), I started in the NHS on the appointed day in 1948. The practice was conducted from a corner terraced house and my wife and I lived upstairs "above the shop". In those days the doctor's wife was an integral part of the practice, acting as unpaid receptionist, telephonist and chaperone. She negotiated with the patients at all hours of the day and night, 24 hours a day and seven days a week. Nearly all GPs were singlehanded and briskly competing with one another.

GPs' workloads were rising, however, and self-preservation prompted the local doctors to organise the Ilford rota scheme which gave us time off for half days and weekends. An employed agent ran it from his house with patients phoning a central number. We split into five groups to cover each other's patients in a roster of one in ten. We also agreed to stagger our holidays and when I or my colleagues were away, the remaining doctors would see our patients. I remember once returning from two weeks' summer vacation and being quickly spotted by lots of patients who chased us, insisting on consultations in the street.

Patients started queuing in the front garden as early as 6 am, some to get in from the cold and many others to get their sick notes for work, especially on a Monday morning. On one infamous occasion an irate patient kicked in the front door in the early hours and ran upstairs to confront myself and wife in bed! Thirty home visits a day was average but during one influenza epidemic I actually did 50 visits over a 24 hour period.

Most GPs attended home confinements, which, in the absence of a reasonable bed, were sometimes conducted on the kitchen table. The local midwife was in attendance. Most were excellent but one I worked with was particularly unpleasant, swearing like a trooper at the patients during labour – a veritable Sarah Gamp.

Patients expected a bottle of medicine

In those days all the GPs dispensed medicine for the patients. Most had been conditioned to expect a bottle and the surgery contained several Winchester flasks of coloured fluids, mostly aspirin and other placebo mixtures, to meet their expectations if not always their medical needs.

I remember my excitement as patients signed on my medical list. Before the NHS, only salaried employees were covered by National Health Insurance; wife and children were not and had to pay to visit the doctor. Not surprisingly, in a working class area they were reluctant to come to the surgery. However, they did not take long after the NHS started to discover that they no longer had to pay. So doctors were inundated, with many patients bringing their previously untreated ailments. One old lady in particular stuck in my mind: she came with a fulminating carcinoma of the breast. Sadly, such tragedies were depressingly common. Eye and dental checks were free and I spent much time filling up green OSCI forms for patients to have eye tests. All this left me in no doubt about the value of the NHS to the community, though the backlog of illness meant hard work for GPs and hospitals.

The only contraception available was condoms and men bought these "secretly" at barbers and some, but by no means all, chemist shops. The social taboos surrounding family planning meant that frequently women asked me to arrange abortions. Before the 1967 Abortion Act, initiated by the Liberal MP David Steel as a Private Member's Bill, this could be done legally only with a psychiatrist's support. So, many women had back street abortions, often with horrible consequences. Steel's legislation saved many women from such horrors.

My experiences in a working class practice prompted me to become involved in female family planning, which in those days consisted of fitting Dutch caps. I subsequently chaired the local family planning clinic and its remit included educating young people. The clinic was, however, frowned upon by the local community, and professions and doctors working in it had to look over their shoulders before entering the premises, a striking contrast to modern attitudes to contraception.

A cottage industry

In the early days general practice was very much a cottage industry, but the therapeutic revolution and many other innovations enabled general

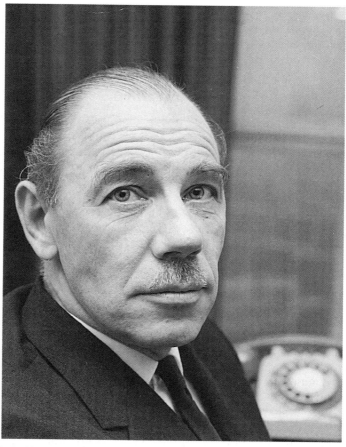

Kenneth Robinson (later Sir) was appointed Minister of Health in Harold Wilson's 1964 Labour Administration. During his time in office he negotiated a new contract for general practitioners with the BMA which was to launch a renaissance in primary care.

46

practice to provide a better service for patients and to move forward from the "knife and fork", singlehanded practice. Many of these innovations were stimulated by the Family Doctors' Charter of 1966, negotiated between the BMA, led by GP Jim Cameron, and the Minister of Health, Kenneth Robinson. Foremost was the introduction of group practice, allowing GPs to share services in purposebuilt or adapted premises. It was, however, difficult for singlehanded GPs to acquire a sufficient number of patients to make their practices financially viable, if they were to provide the service available in group practices. This could be done only in urban areas, by acquiring patients from other doctors or by combining with others.

Forming my group practice took many years of patient negotiation. My first step was to enter into partnership with an older lady doctor, so that when she retired the practice had two surgery premises, enabling us to attract new, young doctors. The next step was to find central premises for the whole practice. This eventually happened when the local authority built a health centre on the campus of the local district hospital.

Another innovation was an appointment system for attendances at surgeries. This not only saved patients having to wait hours to see the doctor, but also helped to spread the load so that the patients did not all come on Mondays and Fridays for their signing on and off sickness certificates. My practice was one of the early ones to introduce such a system. We did it gradually to overcome the patients' suspicions. All my local colleagues were also sceptical, claiming that it could not be done in their practices and obviously I had a different type of patient from them!

Health centres and primary care teams: a changing scenario

The great idea of health centres was to enable the GPs to work with the community services under one roof as a team. Patients would no longer have to go from one building to another looking for help. It was a bold aim but in practice proved difficult to achieve because of the different administrative and financial structures under which the participants operated. GPs were self-employed and under contract to a government agency; community nurses were salaried and employed by the local authority and subsequently health authorities. Social workers also worked for the local authority. In my group the primary care team met every Friday after morning surgery. At its best, it consisted of the GPs, district nurse, health visitor, community psychiatric nurse, clinical psychologist, and social worker. Later, we also had a practice nurse. We discussed the problems of our mutual patients, each professional giving his or her views: this was the primary care team at its best and it did a magnificent job for patients, especially the vulnerable ones.

In order to foster the team work, I had negotiated a unified management structure of all services in the centre. I regret that since I retired from practice the competitive market philosophy has replaced the co-operation there as elsewhere in the NHS.

Now there are five separate practices, each with its own manager, some even employing additional business and fund managers. Each practice has its own receptionists, secretary, and nurse. There is a separate community manager as well as managers of community nurses, the latter working on an area rather than practice basis. Community psychiatric nurses and psychologists have been withdrawn and are now attached to the mental health department; the social worker has departed for an area office. So for possibly twice the price, the patient may be getting only half of the previous excellent service.

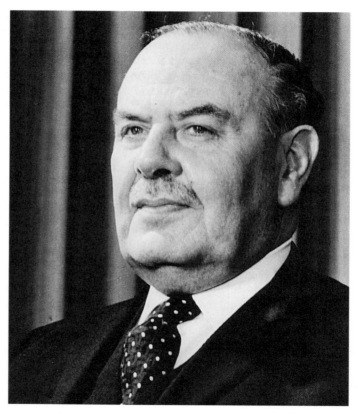

The general practitioners' negotiating team during the mid 60's confrontation with the Labour Government headed by Dr (later Sir) James Cameron. The ussions, based on the profession's *Charter for the Family Doctor Service*, were to be protracted and difficult. Agreement was finally reached in 1966. Reproduced with permission from Getty Images.

I also was involved, on a part-time basis, in a pioneer scheme to improve the quality of primary care. I was the first general practitioner facilitator in the country and worked in the Inner London Borough of Islington, which contains many deprived communities. This work has led to the widespread use of facilitators by health authorities, though now they are not medically qualified. The scheme was a forerunner of the General Medical Council's recently introduced scheme for improving the practice of poorly performing doctors.

I was impressed by how much help an attached social worker could give to patients with personal difficulties. To have her in the same building for face to face discussion with other members of the team was a great advantage. The alternative, unfortunately, is impersonal telephone messages. Regrettably, there was some animosity and misunderstanding about the roles of doctors and social workers. I well remember the then Secretary of State, Sir Keith Joseph, addressing a meeting of the Ilford Medical Society and when asked why patients received so little help from social workers, he replied "That is the responsibility of the local council". The large medical audience rose spontaneously and shouted down the minister. Subsequently, the Director of Social Services spelt out the inadequate resources allocated to her department. While this helped a little to soothe the doctors, it did not help their patients.

Seebohm reforms of social services

Before the Seebohm Inquiry of 1968, which led to radical reforms in social work, social workers had operated as specialists, for example, psychiatric social workers and those in children's departments. The Seebohm Report, which was adopted by the government, introduced the concept of generic social workers. These were generalists and were employed by the local authority under the Director of Social Services, who also took over the duties of the former Children's Officer.

GPs were not happy at losing the skilled support of specialised social workers. Medical social workers had evolved from hospital almoners, a highly regarded profession whose origins lay in the late 19th century. After Seebohm they were no longer health service employees but were administered from local authority offices. This change was resisted in vain by these workers, whose loyalties had previously been to the medical profession: unfortunately, the consequence was some animosity between newly recruited social workers and doctors.

One particular anxiety among doctors has been the question of confidentiality of information on patients because social workers have had an ambivalent relationship with their employers on this subject. The BMA believes the difficulties over confidentiality would be overcome if the government set up a social work council similar to the General Medical

Council. Such a council would have ethical, disciplinary, and educational functions. Education is already catered for by the Central Council for Education and Training for Social Work, but though the idea of a statutory GMC style council is supported by the British Association of Social Workers, the Tory government did not act. The Department of Health also turned down the Central Council's proposal to increase the basic training from two to three years. Perhaps the new Labour government will react more constructively to these overdue reforms, which would improve the status and skills of social work professionals and would, I hope, improve working relations with doctors.

During a professional life spent wholly in the NHS, I have experienced several reorganisations introduced by different governments. Unfortunately, these did not necessarily improve the service for either patients or doctors. Nevertheless, I am convinced that until the past decade the NHS has generally given a reasonable service to the British people and at a bargain price. Indeed, the persistent underfunding has been well publicised but despite this shortage of resources, committed professionals usually managed – at least until the 1990s – to maintain high standards of medical care. That commitment is faltering under the impact of competitive forces unleashed by recent internal market "reforms". These have so changed the service that after 50 years, I , as a senior citizen, am worried that when I am most likely to need the NHS it is but a shadow of the original concept of its founders. I can only hope that the policies of the Labour government will mitigate the damage caused by the 1991 internal market.

8: A fortunate man

Somerled Fergusson

The start of the NHS in 1948 was not so great a professional shock to me as to many others, for I had been born into the Highlands and Islands Medical Service which, predating the NHS by 35 years, embodied many of the new service's features and a few more that have not yet been realised. My father was a singlehanded general practitioner in Ardnamurchan and when his health began to fail (a result of war service), I returned home to assist him. Four years later, at the age of 57, he died suddenly in my arms of a massive coronary thrombosis. Since I had no written partnership agreement with him the executive council appointed an older doctor as his successor and I had to seek another practice. It was a stressful time because I had to find a home for my mother and family, Highlands and Islands practices having "tied" houses.

Naturally I was disappointed but this experience left me with a strong sense of the meaning of justice and a firm resolve to do my utmost for any of my colleagues or their patients should they be disadvantaged and I in a position to help them, and it also motivated me to enter medical politics locally and nationally. Soon afterwards, with the support of Dr Ian Pennie, then LMC Secretary, I was fortunate to be appointed to a practice in Sutherland, which carried with it a seat on the local medical committee (LMC) and subsequently membership of the local executive council. My apprenticeship in medicopolitics then took me through a range of NHS and professional bodies including the Highland Health Board, Scottish Medical Practices Committee, the BMA's Scottish Council and GMSC, and the association's rural subcommittees.

I consider myself a fortunate man to have spent over 40 years in general practice in the Highlands. There were drawbacks – for example, the long distances patients had to travel to hospitals, professional isolation, the burden of providing 24 hour cover, and the difficulties of arranging time off. These were problems which, as I explain later, I tried to mitigate. But overall, I enjoyed general practice. Participating in medicopolitics gave me an insight into the NHS's workings and I have used my experiences as the basis of this personal view of the service's first 50 years.

In 1965, at the time of the negotiations on the Family Doctors' Charter, the Scottish Home and Health Department initiated an inquiry (the Birsay

Committee) "to consider the arrangements for the provision of the general medical services in the Highlands and Islands within the framework of the heath services generally; and to make recommendations". I served on this inquiry, which largely repeated the work of the Dewar Committee, which had instigated the introduction of the Highlands and Islands Medical Service in 1913. Many of the Birsay Committee's recommendations were incorporated in the NHS reorganisation in 1974 and benefited rural practice. With one proposal, however, I disagreed. This was a suggested change in the mileage and inducement arrangements which would have been detrimental for many practices. When entering a minute of reservation, I laid down what a proper remuneration system for general practice in the Highlands and Islands should provide.

- A good standard of medical care and an incentive to improvement.
- Proper premises and equipment.
- An inducement to doctors to come and stay in the Highlands and Islands (the whole area, not just part of it).
- Recognition for the workload, the extent of responsibility, the numbers of population involved, and the area covered.
- A reasonable income for the doctor.

These criteria are as relevant today as when they were written. Sadly, the remuneration system has not been altered and problems have persisted. (The knowledge and information gleaned from this inquiry were to prove invaluable in the future.)

Isolation, distance, and communications

Scotland comprises three eighths of the United Kingdom in area but contains only some 5 million people. My own LMC area (Highland), an eighth of the total at more than 10,000 square miles (larger than Wales), is the most sparsely populated of all. My practice, by no means the largest, covered 700 square miles, reaching halfway across Scotland. So, the usual rural practice problems of isolation, distance, and communications were writ large in the Highland area. In particular, local communities faced severe difficulties in getting prompt emergency care.

To tackle this deficiency in rural care, in 1969 the Health Board set up an inquiry into our accident service chaired by Mr Ian Campbell. This recommended setting up a unified radiocommunications system linking all the contributing services: GPs, nurses, ambulances, fire service, police, hospitals, etc. As Chairman of the Area Medical Committee, I persuaded the Highland Health Board to allocate £104,000 for the first phase. Unfortunately, because some details were confidential, I was unable to convince my colleagues of the scheme's potential in co-ordinating effort and saving time, and the money was lost to other priorities within the NHS.

It was an opportunity lost and in 1995 Sir Thomas Thomson, reporting on *Health Care in Remote and Island Areas in Scotland*, referred to the continuing need for co-ordinated emergency services.

GPs had to undertake several procedures not normally done in those days by family doctors. One such was minor surgery. We had sterilisers but I was never entirely happy with their effectiveness and when in 1978 our central sterile supplies department had spare capacity, the CAMO, Dr Alex Morrison, and I persuaded that department to sterilise small treatment packs, the GPs supplying the instruments. This scheme caught on rapidly, pre-empting the minor surgery components in the 1989 GP contract by a dozen years.

My generation of doctors did not know what physiological changes occurred if seriously injured patients were not stabilised within the first hour, but practical experience taught us that this interval could be critical. Until 1961 my village had no ambulance; that meant a minimum five hour delay in admitting seriously ill or injured patients to hospital. Having exhausted all normal channels in an effort to speed up emergency admissions, I arranged to see my MP, the late Sir David Robertson. I took with me to the House of Commons a list of all emergency admissions over the previous six months with length of time taken and distances covered before the patients received treatment – but no names. Sir David read it, left me listening to a debate and returned in half an hour to say, "I have just been speaking to the Secretary of State. Go home, Fergusson, you will have your ambulance within a fortnight". True to his word a six month old Morris ambulance was soon delivered: I can still recall the registration number – 475 AJA. Those were the days when GPs were listened to and MPs really were a power for good and not just parliamentary "lobby fodder". Our new ambulance meant that patients could then reach hospital in three hours, but that was still too long.

Air ambulance service

Thanks to an enterprising GP, Dr A.J. MacLeod, the Highlands and Islands had benefited from an air ambulance service since the early 1930s. Unfortunately, however, 25 years on large areas still had no suitable landing grounds. When a great snowstorm cut off the Highlands in 1955 the Royal Navy based an aircraft carrier, HMS Glory, in Loch Eriboll. Using her as a staging post, the Fleet Air Arm flew doctors and their patients, myself included, around the area in the old Whirlwind helicopters. Operation Snowdrop, as it was named, proved so successful that the Health Department was petitioned to provide a permanent helicopter ambulance service. Reluctantly, the government agreed to the use of service planes in emergencies. But finally in 1990, after a successful pilot scheme in Tayside (sponsored by British Telecom), the Scottish Home and Health Department set up the Helicopter Ambulance Service, based at Raigmore Hospital. Thus most people in the Highlands and Islands were brought within one hour's flying time of a hospital. At last, we had achieved the "magic hour". But it had taken years of perseverance to do so.

So much for ambulance cases: there remained the "walking wounded" and those patients attending clinics. They had to make their own way with minimal public transport, often at inappropriate times. This was very costly for patients travelling a long distance and a disincentive to obtaining adequate treatment. I thought this was unfair and urged the late George McIver, Chairman of Sutherland Executive Council and Vice Chairman of the Northern Regional Hospital Board, to obtain official approval for patients from outlying areas to have their travelling expenses refunded, less the first £1. The latter would, I thought, discourage abuse and restrict the scheme to the Highlands and Islands but the bureaucrats imposed a 30 mile limit before patients could receive benefit, a restriction which immediately created anomalies. Not surprisingly, patients' contributions are now much higher. Even so, it is a worthwhile service for communities, most of whose members are not well off.

A "fairly free hand"

When I was elected to chair the Scottish Rural Practice Subcommittee, Dr Keith Davidson, the SGMSC Chairman, gave me a "fairly free hand" to further the interests of Scottish rural doctors and their patients, but obviously within the constraints of the profession as a whole. This also gave me a seat on the Rural Practices Subcommittee (UK). In London I tried to foster good relations between rural GPs in Scotland and those elsewhere by giving my UK chairman my unwavering support, even though the main concerns of English and Welsh rural doctors were dispensing arrangements whereas ours were with mileage and inducement payments. This loyalty was later repaid handsomely. During this time, I worked to improve the contract for doctors in the inducement scheme. Some progress was made. Though not all changes were quantifiable in cash terms, taken together they represented tangible improvement in the lot of this group spread over time, though not all of them were able to appreciate this.

Remedies for professional isolation

Membership of the Scottish Medical Practices Committee (SMPC) enabled me to encourage the introduction of an extra 20 principals into the Highland area and many more into the rest of rural Scotland. This allowed many practices to be double manned, thus relieving to some extent doctors' isolation. The SMPC had a formula for assessing the need for extra doctors, with a special dispensation for those (mainly women) who "for domestic or other reasons were not freely mobile". On one occasion I enjoyed turning this principle on its head, by getting it applied to a young male doctor who was tied to an area because his wife was a teacher, invoking what, with tongue in cheek, I called the "Indiscriminate Sex Act". Even so, many singlehanded doctors still worked in isolation because the new arrangement could not be applied to them even though we managed to introduce two and three doctor inducement practices where the service was classed as "essential". Though the formula could justify the need it did not bring any extra funding, a not uncommon outcome in the NHS. Furthermore, though the Family Doctors' Charter had rescued general practice as a whole in the UK, it actually worked to the financial detriment of a section of Scottish rural practice, a deficiency that has yet to be rectified.

What of the future?

For me, the NHS ceased to exist on 1 April 1991. It was replaced by a business oriented, price motivated organisation myopically focused on "single column accounting" and incapable of taking a broad view. I have worked all my life in a caring service and this mercenary approach scunners me, especially where it adversely affects the elderly.

No wonder morale is so low, but health professionals are resilient and have overcome upheavals before. They will do so again. So I end with this toast to my successors:

> There is but a past for me,
> The future lies ahead of thee,
> Be therefore of good cheer you see,
> The best is yet to be.

The Scottish rural practices subcommittee was determined to help those doctors who despite the changes were still isolated. So "Mac" Armstrong (my successor in the chair of the Scottish Rural Practices Subcommittee, now Secretary of the BMA) and I produced a scheme to provide those smaller practices not helped by the "formula" or inducement schemes with an Assistant (Associate) shared between two or three such practices. It was based on the old Highlands and Islands Assistant/Successor scheme and would be funded centrally. Fortunately, David Farrow, then Chairman of the UK subcommittee, handsomely repaid my earlier loyalty by ensuring that this item stayed on the negotiating agenda.

Nothing came of this, however, until March 1987 when the Chairman of the Highland Health Board asked me (as a board member) to review the position. Seizing the opportunity, I presented my report, which came to be called the "Highland Review", two months later. James McWilliam, the Chairman, all credit to him, breached his terms of reference by taking an item concerning terms and conditions of service of GPs to the Minister of State on the grounds that it affected *patients*. It then became a *board* initiative and the rest is history. The Associate Scheme, however, had to wait for the introduction of the new GP contract in 1989 since it required "new" money, the first since the Charter. No one, wherever they practise, now has to be isolated because this Highlands and Islands scheme created the precedent for a variety of other assistant type arrangements (the first in Liverpool) and formed the framework for job sharing, part-time principals, etc.

In an organisation as extensive as the NHS no single individual's involvement can encompass the whole and any observations of mine must be purely personal dependent on an ageing memory of events. I have been fortunate to have lived through such interesting times and feel privileged, with the help of many others too numerous to name, to have particpated, albeit in a minor way, in shaping events.

9: The first 50 years: a basic guide to cost, activity, and manpower changes

Jon Ford

During its 50 year existence the NHS has undergone numerous transformations. These have often made it difficult to compare past and present figures of cost, activity, and personnel. Geographical consistency is difficult to achieve and successive reorganisations and changes in definitions have obscured often significant trends. Nevertheless, I offer the following comparisons to help put into context the contributions to this volume.

Cost

Expenditure on the NHS in 1949–1950 totalled £447 million for the UK. This represented a little under 4% of gross domestic product (GDP) at the time. Expenditure in 1996–1997 by comparison was a massive £42,987 million or nearly 6% of GDP. A sizeable proportion of this nearly 100-fold growth is of course accounted for by inflation. On the basis of the broadest measure of background inflation (the so-called GDP deflator), NHS expenditure in 1996–1997 was still some £2266 million at 1949–1950 prices – a fivefold increase. Even now, however, the NHS absorbs a considerably smaller proportion of gross domestic product than public health expenditure in many of its European neighbours (Table 9.1). It has of course long spent less on total health care – state and private sectors – than most of them.

Expenditure on the hospital and community health services accounts for the bulk of total, as it did originally. Its share of the total, allowing for changed coverage, has remained fairly static, rising from around 58% of total to 62% over the period since 1948. Expenditure on general medical services has lost share from around 11% to just over 8%, while the share going to the pharmaceutical service has increased from 8% to around 12%. Capital expenditure has doubled its share of hospital and community health service expenditure from 2·4% in 1949–1950 to just under 5% today. It

Table 9.1   Total and state expenditure on health as a percentage of GDP (1995)

Country	Total health spending as % of GDP	State health spending as % of GDP
Austria	7·9	5·9
Belgium	8·0	7·0
Denmark	6·4	5·3
France	9.8	7·7
Germany	10.4	8·2
Greece	5·8	4·4
Ireland	6·4	5·1
Italy	7·7	5·4
Luxemburg	7·0	6·5
Netherlands	8·8	6·8
Norway	8·0	6·6
Portugal	8·2	5·0
Spain	7·6	6·0
Sweden	7·2	5·9
United Kingdom	6·9	5·9

now represents annual expenditure of around £2 billion. Since the beginning of the health service, there has been enormous investment in premises by general practitioners, underpinned by the cost and notional rent schemes introduced in the 1960s. Payments under these schemes now total some £150 million annually, representing an estimated £2 billion of capital assets.

Activity

Changes in total expenditure and in share of total do not fully reflect the quite dramatic changes that the NHS has undergone in the past 50 years. The numbers of hospital beds occupied daily have fallen by nearly half (220,000 in England and Wales as against 400,000 in 1949–1950), while the throughput of the service after allowance for changed definition has increased from 3 million to 10 million inpatients per year. Over the same period, the growth in the population has been only 19%. Significantly, of 11·3 million finished consultant episodes in 1995–1996, 22% were day cases. Activity has also dramatically increased for outpatients, new cases now totalling 11 million as against 6 million in 1949–1950, total attendances having grown from 26 to 40 million. The growth in share of total expenditure of the pharmaceutical services manifests itself in an increase in prescriptions per head of population from less than five in 1949–1950, to eight today. The growth also reflects the substantial increase in the number of prescribable drugs available and the high cost of some of them.

The workforce

The NHS is one of the largest employers in the world with currently just over 1 million employees and contractors. This is roughly double the number at the inception of the NHS. The largest single staff group is nursing staff. There are now some 440,000 nurses and midwives employed in the NHS compared with 190,000 in 1950; however, the numbers of nurses are falling and over half a million were employed in the late 1980s. Skill mix within the NHS workforce is changing in response to structural and clinical changes, one example being the transfer of some clinical and record keeping duties from junior doctors to clinical nurses. Skill mix changes are likely to continue, and some hospital activities may be transferred to primary health care teams in the community.

Doctors

At the start of the NHS, there were 48,000 doctors in active practice in Great Britain, of which 17,000 were general practitioners and 29,000 were hospital doctors. This represented approximately one doctor per 1000 inhabitants. Today there are nearly 107,000 doctors in active practice or one per 550 inhabitants (Table 9.2). A steadily rising proportion of them are women as the number of women graduating annually as doctors has for several years exceeded 50% of total medical graduates and in 1995 31% of GPs in England (including assistants and trainees) were women.

Table 9.2   Estimated total of active doctors 1995 (UK)

	1995
Hospital doctors	61,050
Public health medicine	1127
Community health	2011
General practice	34,594
Total NHS	98,782
Non-NHS	8072
Total active doctors	**106,854**

10:   Regions: dead and buried or hope for resurrection?

Malcolm Forsythe

At a recent function at the Royal College of Physicians, I was chatting to a retired consultant who had been a non-executive member of a regional health authority. He discussed their abolition. He commented how only a few years ago his regional chairman had told the health authority that the Secretary of State for Health had assured him personally that regions would always be safe. The chairman had reinforced this assurance by adding that it would be political suicide for any government to get rid of them.

Well, it has happened and my key question is whether health care will be affected. But first, why were they ever created? Back in 1920, Lord Dawson of Penn sent the then Minister of Health, Mr Addison, an interim report on the future provision of health and allied services on behalf of the Consultative Council on Medical and Allied Services. That report, in remarkably clear detail, identified three levels of care in what were called "health centres". These can be considered as analogous to today's primary, secondary and tertiary care, with the latter being located within under-graduate teaching hospitals on the basis that "the teaching hospital would receive cases of unusual difficulty and those (patients) requiring specialised knowledge or equipment".

During the debates in Parliament on the National Health Service Bill in 1946, the question as to whether to have regionally organised hospital services loomed large. The Nuffield Provincial Hospitals Trust had become an active protagonist of regions as a result of the very careful survey it had undertaken of hospitals within the United Kingdom during the Second World War. In the end – and after a fierce Cabinet battle between Home Secretary Herbert Morrison, proponent of a local authority based health service, and Aneurin Bevan, the Minister for Health – regional hospital boards were created in 1948. Every board had at least one medical school within its geographical area and England initially had 13 boards, rising to 14 with the later creation of the Wessex region.

I qualified 13 years after the NHS started. During that time financial pressures had steadily worsened. Inadequate capital stock, greater than expected patients' needs, staff pay demands and rising costs for drugs, dental, and eye care figured prominently among the causes. Indeed, within two years of the service's launch the Labour government had initiated an inquiry into the widening gap between cost estimates for and actual spending on the NHS. As the financial conduit between central government and hospitals, regional boards were in the thick of the battles over funds. The boards employed and deployed all senior medical staff (other than hospitals with boards of governors), allocated capital for medical and surgical equipment as well as new fabric and allotted revenue to the hospital management committees (HMC). The financial responsibilities were onerous but these gave them power as the main agents of change for the hospital services.

Some 23 years on from the NHS's foundation the US Senate Health Subcommittee led by its Chairman, Senator Edward Kennedy, came to study the NHS. Though they found much to criticise, the senator and his colleagues described the improvement in the geographical distribution of high quality specialist services as a great achievement. Furthermore, the subcommittee observed that the strong primary care services allowed specialists to concentrate on their own particular skills. "It was for this reason," the report stated, "that the British could manage with fewer neurosurgeons than there were in the city of San Francisco."

Enthusiasm for regionalised care

During the 1970s a wave of enthusiasm spread across the developed countries for the introduction of regionalised medical care. In 1975 the Milbank Memorial Fund reproduced the whole of the 1920 Dawson Report as part of a publication on *The Regionalization of Personal Medical Services*. In the same book, Kerr White described three types of epidemiological problems:

> Firstly, there are problems that have a high probability of affecting each of us several times in the course of a lifetime, such as gastrointestinal infections, musculoskeletal problems, emotional problems, etc., and they occupy the time of one practitioner for every 2,000 to 3,000 people. Second, there are problems that require a population of perhaps twenty-five thousand to a couple of hundred thousand for efficient provision of care. These are problems like cardiac failure, common fractures, abdominal surgery, and so on; they require a second level of care, a second level of knowledge and technology and facilities. Third, there are problems that require populations of perhaps a half million to a million or so to generate sufficient numbers to really occupy and maintain the skills of the tertiary care levels, the supporting staff, and the necessary technological facilities and equipment.

Kerr White concluded by saying that "The principal reason for region-alization, if one attempts to invoke science or rational calculations, is getting the right kinds of personnel and the right kinds of knowledge to tackle these patient problems, given their distribution".

In the United Kingdom the resources to build, equip and run necessary new hospitals were slow to materialise compared with other Western countries. The pattern of district general hospitals across the nation, proposed in 1962 by the then Minister of Health, Enoch Powell, was designed to provide around ten beds per 1000 population. Later, in 1969, the Bonham Carter Report on the functions of the district general hospital recommended that these beds should be provided in hospitals with around 2000 beds so as to ensure that economies of scale were achieved and that no consultant worked in isolation. Hence it was nicknamed "The Noah's Ark Report". In the event other government priorities (for example, Secretary of State Barbara Castle's "people before buildings" policy and the energy crisis) delayed most of these schemes, except where other independent sources of capital were available, for instance in London teaching hospitals. Regions had to develop innovative plans to accommodate the increasing demand for secondary care. These plans included day hospitals, home dialysis, domino maternity delivery, hospital at home, the hospice movement, and greater use of well placed general practitioner hospitals.

Consolidation of regions

Regions, whether in the shape of regional hospital boards or regional health authorities, in their efforts to improve the distribution of specialist services also needed to redistribute capital and revenue. The Resource Allocation Working Party (RAWP) Report in 1976 created the mechanism for this redistribution. At that time some of the most hostile board and health authority meetings were provoked by the process of reallocating resources. The value of regions as a buffer between the Secretary of State and those responsible for providing specialist services became apparent. Reallocation was necessary not only geographically within regions but also between different care groups. Several formal inquiries had shown that the NHS was neglecting the mentally ill, as well as those suffering from learning disabilities. Regions were ideally placed to mastermind the closure of the large institutions caring for these people and to provide the appropriate local services across a large number of districts. The creation of a bipartite structure in 1974 by the integration of hospital and community health services seemed at the time to consolidate the position of regions. Furthermore, regions were also responsible for the appointment and resourcing of the newly established community health councils – the first official acknowledgement of the so-called consumer voice.

The 1980s saw a dramatic rise in the need for investment in skills, equipment, and cash for a whole range of regional diagnostic and treatment services. These included transplantation, neonatal intensive care, forensic psychiatry, and genetics. Most regions developed collaborative contractual arrangements with the designated providers, as did the Department of Health for the supraregional specialist services. The perennial problem of insufficient resources persisted but in my experience was recognised by all participants. Needs assessment, prioritisation, and evaluation were all part of the negotiating process and as a regional medical officer, one of my essential functions was to ensure that negotiations took account of the medical dimension.

Regions were not, however, just concerned with service matters. The health service always had significant responsibilities for major training and continuing education. Postgraduate deans were appointed in the 1960s and always worked closely with the senior administrative medical officers and their successors. Regions also developed major research initiatives concentrating on biomedical subjects but increasingly incorporating research into the delivery of health services. Not surprisingly, therefore, when the Department of Health wanted to strengthen research and development each regional authority was asked to appoint its own director of research and development. So by 1990 regional authorities, with their three principal functions of service planning and resource allocation, training and continuing education, and research and development all properly established, seemed ideally structured to lead the NHS into the future.

The senior administrative medical officers of 1948 became regional medical officers in 1974 and then regional directors of public health in 1988. Their influence on the service was enormous but their authority was always dependent on their maintaining the trust and confidence of the medical profession within the region, often after unpalatable choices had been made. The principal forum was the statutory medical advisory committee but among many other key power points were the regional postgraduate medical and manpower committees. The relationship with university medical schools was also critical. The late Sir William Trethowan fondly recalled his weekly meetings, when dean, with the regional medical officer, after which "things just happened".

Death of the regions

The Thatcher government launched its radical reform of the NHS with *Working for Patients* in 1989. Regional health authorities' responsibilities for strategic planning were clearly at an end so it was natural that the government should first cut their number and eventually abolish them. This happened in April 1996. I see it as paradoxical that while on the one hand regions lost their important service responsibilities, on the other, the need for research and development and postgraduate medical and dental education to be regionally organised became even more prominent. If

63

today's postgraduate deans and regional directors of research and development working within the new civil service style regional offices are wise, they will retain their university locus. The creation of trusts also meant that consultants were no longer regional employees and thus their enthusiasm for collaborative decisions on the distribution of services vanished into the NHS market place.

The future

I foresee that:

- whatever politicians may claim, the NHS will suffer further changes;
- attempts to achieve rationalisation of clinical services by merging trusts or combining health authorities will achieve limited success;
- squabbles between the health and social services over care responsibilities will increase, prompting suggestions for merging health with local government;
- such a change would, among other consequences, further distance ministers from the firing line;
- health professionals will suffer greater pressures from ever rising public expectations, more and more complaints and litigation, and the need to demonstrate regularly competence and good performance;
- medicine will, however, remain a wonderful vocation and medical leadership of hospital and community trusts will evolve naturally.

Why have we thrown away a structure that was once the envy of other nations? The reasons are probably legion but, over time, these have had a cumulative effect. It was always going to be an uphill task while the regions were quangos, neither physically nor functionally coterminous with any other public services, not even with any of the utilities. Their limited political influence was reduced further as board and authority membership moved from one of unpaid representatives from all parts of the NHS and walks of life to a handful of non-executives appointed by the Secretary of State for Health and rewarded financially. For example, the South East Metropolitan Regional Hospital Board went from 23 members in 1972 – which included an MP, two county councillors, two borough councillors, a university vice chancellor, a medical school dean, six other doctors, a nurse, and a trade union representative – to six non-executives at the time of its abolition, with only the university slot surviving. Admittedly, boards' links with local government were always tenuous and the latter had their own headaches coping with financial cutbacks and restructuring. Even so, how different matters might have been had regional local government been introduced.

Regions must also take some blame for being far too complacent and occasionally plain incompetent. The Hospital (then Health) Advisory

Service and the Audit Commission evolved from circumstances where regions had failed to monitor the operation of services adequately and/or to invest equitably. When in the 1980s two regions spectacularly squandered money on information services which they themselves were managing I feared for the future of the regional structure.

As if that was not enough, regions failed to make their case for continued existence on the basis of their value in providing good medical services. A bulletin on *Effective Health Care 1996* from the NHS Centre for Reviews and Dissemination dealt with "hospital volume and health care outcomes, costs and patient access". It shows how much of the research undertaken has been done outside the UK. Just because the regionalisation of health care made sense in relation to the distribution and treatment of diseases, it did not mean that this effectiveness should not have been demonstrated objectively. Sadly, the necessary research has been done without a benchmark, so it will be impossible to measure any effects on health care following the regions' abolition.

Will regions return? I believe that 50 years on from their creation they still make medical, management, and community sense. Indeed, health authorities today have formed consortia or made other collaborative arrangements to ensure they plan and purchase tertiary services sensibly. Future mergers of these authorities could end up with bodies responsible for populations comparable in size to the previous smaller regions. The newly elected Labour administration might well restructure local government. If so, we could get regionally elected bodies with planning and resource allocation responsibilities embracing social services, education and the environment. It would then be logical to add health responsibilities. Perhaps the Whitehall turf wars that started in the Labour Cabinet of 1946 would finally be ended – to the benefit of patients and staff. We can only wait and hope.

11: Experiences and future visions of the NHS: a younger doctor's perspective

Ruth Gilbert

I qualified as a doctor 15 years ago, yet even from my "younger perspective" my most striking impression of the NHS is of enormous change, both as an organisation and within my own specialty of paediatrics. General management, NHS trusts and purchasers, a reduction in junior doctors' hours and the creation of a unified training grade are just a few of the organisational changes. In paediatric practice, examples include changes in neonatal morbidity brought about by the widespread use of steroids in preterm labour and surfactant; the reduction in invasive *Haemophilus influenzae* infection, which is now so rare that every case is of national interest; the change in incidence of cot death, which reached a peak and then fell by more than 50% simply by putting babies on their backs; and the rise of HIV infection in children which, provided women are offered prenatal testing, is destined to fall substantially.

One surprising element of these changes is the contrast between the driving forces for organisational change—largely political or management ideology—compared with changes in practice, some of which, at least, have been driven by advances in scientific knowledge. Given that the pace of change is likely to accelerate and certainly will not slow down, my hope for the future is that scientific knowledge will be used much more to shape practice in the NHS and to improve its organisation.

But how can the NHS organise for the future when we do not yet know what the new knowledge or technologies will be? What is needed is an NHS which can respond appropriately to scientific advances. However, the prerequisites for achieving this goal are complex. Where scientific evidence is incontrovertible and desired changes are clear, the NHS can make use of protocols or guidelines combined with the "management of change" skills developed over more than a decade of NHS general management. But

66

incontrovertible scientific evidence is rare and even evidence which stands up to methodological scrutiny and gives unequivocal results may not give clearcut answers about what should be done in practice. In reality, most clinical and policy decisions are based on evidence of varying degrees of uncertainty, which is unlikely to be diminished by future scientific advance. The more we know about options for interventions and about the potential for benefiting or harming patients or for increasing or reducing costs, the more complex are the decisions about who could or should benefit. Most often, scientific evidence needs to be interpreted in the light of practical experience, what matters most to individual patients, and what is feasible within the health care system.

NHS dependent on the "thinking clinician"

So who are the interpreters and integrators of science into practice in the NHS? In my view, the NHS has been and always will be dependent on the "thinking clinician" to make judgements about the appropriate integration of scientific advances into practice. I believe that the development of a science based NHS needs to take place on three fronts.

- Strengthen the body of robust and clinically relevant scientific evidence.
- Focus on how the NHS as an organisation can better nurture the "thinking clinician".
- Promote debate and questioning within the NHS, so that "thinking clinicians" are continually required to justify and review their judgements: this will keep clinicians receptive to the accelerating pace of scientific advance and give broad consideration to the appropriateness of changes.

Much needs to be done to generate robust scientific evidence to drive changes in the NHS and I hope that the recent impetus given to clinical and health services research will continue to gain momentum in the next half century. Unfortunately, my experience of the NHS is that much more could be done to nurture the "thinking clinician" and to promote debate. In my view, the products of the work environment and evaluation are at least as important as scientific evidence for the development of an appropriately science responsive NHS.

But first, let me give some practical examples from my experiences as a junior doctor in the early 1980s which highlight how working conditions, elements of the career structure, and education diminished my desire to question and debate practice – in other words, to be a "thinking clinician".

1 It is 3 am and I'm seeing a family with a young child who is said to have fallen out of bed and banged his head. I'm so tired and I'm searching for the energy to be able to convey respect and sympathy but at the same time make sure to get consent for the child to be admitted and gain some clue as to whether this

is a case of child abuse. I just want to admit the child and sort it out in the morning (or get someone else to). My abiding memory of this occasion, and many others, is anger at my working conditions. I worked 84 hours or more on average a week, which made me tired and irritated by this family and restricted me to short term goals, such as getting back to bed as quickly as possible, rather than trying to find out what had really happened to this child.

2 I've been up all night on the neonatal intensive care unit, apart from an hour in bed. Too many sick babies to look after and I didn't manage to take all the routine blood samples before the morning handover. My fellow senior house officer, who has Saturday and Sunday to look forward to on the unit, shows only anger at what I might leave for him, not sympathy for my bad night. His might be worse. No support for colleagues, just self-defence. I stay and finish the work.

3 And then those awful ward rounds when questions are fired about the haemoglobin result or what I hoped to achieve by requesting an X-ray or, worse, why I hadn't done one. I learned to do the same myself as I became more senior. A technique for deflecting attention from my opinion and to give me time to think. Questions to fend off others rather than to expose important gaps in knowledge which might really affect the decisions we make.

These and other experiences left me amazed by the way the working environment could isolate doctors. Numbed by pressure of work from the desire to inquire and trapped between the patient, the next person up the medical hierarchy, and the nurses (who could be supporters or formidable opponents), unable to admit ignorance, fear or tiredness. But I did have other experiences which showed me how teams of clinicians could be supportive and provide excellent training, allow juniors to take clinical responsibility and learn from experience but call for help when needed. And sometimes, ward rounds, X-ray conferences or other clinical meetings did turn out to be opportunities to ask the important naive questions, to debate the evidence and check out what other clinicians considered to be appropriate, rather than opportunities for "point scoring".

Tired doctors are unsafe

I became involved in the campaign to reduce junior doctors' hours of work. The message for the media was simple: tired doctors are unsafe. But for me it was broader than that. I felt that reducing hours was also an important lever to bring more experienced doctors closer to direct patient care and encourage consultants to work together in teams rather than to continue with hierarchies of juniors topped by single consultants, a tradition stretching back to the start of the NHS. I hoped that more horizontal clinical teams would increase the debate about clinical practice, that differences in practice would be questioned more often, that doctors would be more likely to have to justify their actions to colleagues and, possibly, to their patients, and that such informal accountability might improve care.

Gradually, however, I realised that the immediate working environment is just one of a complex set of organisational factors which affect the way clinicians think about their practice. Another factor is the medical profession's outdated career structure, in which intolerance of atypical career patterns and the dependence on patronage encourages "me too" promotions and discourages a heterogeneity of views and debate. It is a tradition that has seriously disadvantaged the career progress of many women doctors, who now comprise more than half the doctors graduating every year in the UK. Perhaps the most important factor, however, is the role played by medical education in the development of a culture of dogma rather than debate. In my experience, undergraduate education mostly consisted of digesting and regurgitating facts with no incentive or strategies for asking and answering questions. For many years after I qualified, I was left with the sense that there were "right" answers that someone knew, but not me. Not until I moved into clinical research in the late 1980s did I learn how much of practice is open to question and how few "right" answers there are.

Suggested steps towards a science based NHS

- Increase the body of clinically relevant, scientific evidence.
- Promote the expectation that science should play a much greater part in shaping practice and the organisation of the NHS.
- Build on existing models of questioning and debate and encourage more explicit justification of the evidence on which clinical and policy decisions are based.
- Clinical teams should be organised with the aim of promoting a culture of questioning and debate.
- Medical education at all levels should generate strategies for asking and answering questions about commonly accepted practice and understanding of the underlying principles in the evaluation of clinical practice.
- The NHS must encourage and facilitate links between researchers and clinicians which promote collaborative, robust, and relevant research.
- Closer co-operation between researchers, clinicians, and managers would facilitate a strategic approach to planning and operating the nation's health services.

Researchers and clinicians need each other

I stayed in research as a clinical epidemiologist. My priorities now relate to the generation of scientific evidence. But I am constantly aware of how much researchers (like me) need clinicians and vice versa. "Thinking clinicians" are essential to identify priority issues to be addressed by research, consider how findings will be applied in practice, and lead to changes in practice. On the other hand, research evidence sufficiently robust to change practice is most efficiently generated by large scale studies requiring collaboration between research methodologists and clinicians. This generates a tension which future researchers, academics, and clinicians – and managers as well – need to address. How do we improve links between the clinical and research communities in order to enhance the clinical relevance of the research agenda, harness and encourage inquiry by "thinking clinicians" through involvement in research, and efficiently generate robust research findings through well designed, large scale studies? And we should not forget the managers: they must understand the value of these links and facilitate their development. One unwelcome consequence of the internal market has been that short term financial objectives have undermined strategic planning and the co-operation between clinical practice, research and medical education that, though not perfect, has been a significant feature of the NHS.

In summary, prerequisites for a science based NHS are "thinking clinicians" and a culture of questioning and debate. Both are required to drive a series of complex interrelationships between scientific research, the work environment, career structure, the education system, and the health care provided for patients. This needs a culture of co-operation operating within a strategic NHS framework.

12: From LCC to NHS: a physician's transition

Alan Gilmour

My uncle, John Howard Simmons, was a physician, the son of a South Norwood GP, who qualified at King's College Hospital, London in 1923. He soon obtained specialist qualifications and a brilliant consultant career seemed his destiny. His health, however, was poor: as a doctor's son his appendicitis had unfortunately been referred to the great Arbuthnot Lane. A surgeon who believed that the Almighty had made a bad job of human bowels, he tried to remedy this by removing as much as he could, particularly the transverse colon. Life with an internal ileostomy had its drawbacks and in time my uncle's adhesions took their toll. Thus the young physician opted for the mundane but more secure (and pensionable) career of medical officer with the London County Council (LCC) hospital service.

As a schoolboy in the 1930s I visited his household during school holidays, watching a career progress through appointments at different LCC hospitals around London. Mostly soundly built but depressingly designed Victorian institutions, these housed thriving, largely self-sufficient communities.

These communities were feudal but of a type based on mutual loyalty and trust. The senior figure was that of the Medical Superintendent, whose patriarchal role was balanced by that of the often daunting mother figure, the Matron. While the Superintendent's was the senior post, the balance of power often reflected respective strengths of personality; one or two hospitals were noted matriarchies. The ruling triumvirate was completed by the Steward, a less dominant but essential administrator of supplies and services. County Hall provided the overall management of the hospital service and also a range of back-up facilities through its specialist departments. Interestingly, the central back-up was a facet of hospital management that went unnoticed when the NHS took over. Not until lifts and other essential equipment began to fail did the new managers notice the absence of the LCC's programmed maintenance services and have to devise their own systems *de novo*.

71

To me, the characteristic of the LCC hospitals was their great camaraderie, even greater during the war with the bombing of London. Each hospital was a compact bustling village, with ordered hierarchies of people valued as individuals with interrelated roles. The doctors may have been the squirearchy but interdependence was a recognised fact of life and socially as well as professionally, examples of mutual support abounded.

Within the hospitals the medical hierarchy was a broad brotherhood as doctors moved around the LCC hospitals, working their way from junior to senior resident MOs up to the top appointments of Medical Superintendent. All were salaried permanent posts and service spirit was strong. By 1939 my uncle was deputy superintendent at St Charles' Hospital, Ladbroke Grove.

Gothic turrets in Kensington back streets

St Charles' was in a depressing North Kensington cul de sac, though the main hospital's turreted Gothic pavilions added a touch of style. Apart from a sparkling new redbrick nurses' home beside the tennis courts, construction was uniformly of drab yellow brick under slate roofs. The hospital was dominated by a huge central tower. It was to be long after the 1948 takeover before there were any substantial structural changes. Indeed, St Charles' was typical of much of Britain's traditional hospital stock, outdated and with its fabric distressed by wartime neglect. But the staff did their utmost to overcome these physical handicaps.

Early in the war my father was captured by the Japanese, my mother was marooned in Australia, and my uncle became my guardian so I stayed in London and lived with him for 12 years until, following in his footsteps, I was a student at King's College Hospital. At St Charles' I was an accepted member of the community, making friends with key people like the hospital engineer and the gate porters who, with their prodigious memory for faces, regulated all entry through the sole entrance gate. These porters were a special breed, alert, cheerful, busy, the main stem of the hospital grapevine and resourceful in any unexpected situation.

The hospital took war in its stride. Younger staff went to the armed forces, and older ones came out of retirement. Beds were allocated for civilian casualties and contingencies made for wounded servicemen. The resourcefulness of matrons, housekeepers, engineers – and gate porters – manifested itself in new ways and the comradeship, if anything, was greater than before. People mattered. Wives mattered, too, and contributed to the social life.

Readers may wonder at my focus on scenes from London's pre-NHS hospitals. There are two reasons. Firstly, as a reminder of the "estates" problems posed for the infant NHS by an enormous backlog of ageing capital stock. The NHS has never overcome this flawed inheritance.

Secondly, on the "human resources" front, an essential component of "service" has been lost. I have been saddened to see hospital staffs' commitment, mutual loyalty, and purpose slowly eroded by the NHS. Slowly, because while old hands were still around some of the old ways stayed with them. But as the NHS took over and developed, I witnessed the social fabric disintegrate; wives were excluded from the hospital scene and social functions which had brought people together, such as local GPs and junior medical staff, became management jamborees without much purpose. Loyalties were divided: a ward sister accustomed to managing her domestic staff found that she had to communicate her needs to a senior nursing officer at another hospital, who would contact the domestic supervisor somewhere else, who would in turn inform domestic staff. The focus on patients and staff collegiality went. Doctors ceased to belong to a cohesive group, becoming rootless nomads attached to successive minor fiefdoms.

Clinical freedom

A common criticism of the pre-NHS local authority hospitals was that doctors lacked clinical freedom. Thus, one of the great anathemas of doctors in the early NHS was the concept of a medical superintendent. This smacked, it was said, of clinical dictatorship, though I was never aware of frustration on this score within the LCC. The superintendent and his deputy were senior surgeon and physician (or vice versa) and certainly they contributed clinical experience, but their management, as I saw it, was one of resources. The tasks allotted to medical staff could be altered to cope with the needs of the moment. At St Charles' I can remember my uncle coming home to lunch one day in unfamiliar surgical garb – there was a run on "Ts & As" (tonsils and adenoids), the wholesale removal of which was a feature of those pre-antibiotic days–and it was a case of "all hands to the theatres". I used to wonder if the cries of interference with clinical freedom, if valid at all, were more relevant to the superintendents of the old mental asylums. One of the NHS's greatest achievements was to provide a good specialist service nationwide. But the LCC had maintained a panel of distinguished specialists who could be called in consultation over difficult cases–"honoraries" as they were then called from their unpaid appointments at teaching hospitals. In about 1943, however, the LCC introduced their own full-time consultant posts and my uncle was one of the first successful applicants, being appointed consultant physician to Lewisham Hospital, a general hospital whose catchment area included a population of over 300,000.

So we moved from the spacious Victorian house at St Charles', where we had lived through the worst of the "blitz", to Blackheath in time for the flying bombs or V1s, followed closely by the V2 supersonic rockets.

Experience of organising the hospital for wartime needs, including secret planning for use of beds for anticipated military casualties, was something my uncle put to good use in later years. One flying bomb glided silently into the crowded shopping centre at Woolworth's in Lewisham one Saturday and again it was "all hands to the theatres".

When the NHS took over there were probably fewer immediate changes at Lewisham than at many other hospitals. My uncle soon inherited the role of Superintendent in what must have been a totally *ad hoc* arrangement made by the hospital management committee. While officially the senior full-time consultant physician, he also acted in an honorary management capacity that was to serve the hospital well. This was not so everywhere: the new *gauleiter* at one hospital where I later worked railroaded the Medical Superintendent out of his house so fast he had to slaughter all his hens, although he stayed on as a physician. My uncle told me with a quiet grin that he and his secretary were always a good three weeks ahead of the formal decision making processes of the official secretariat, who occupied a full floor of offices overhead. The LCC had helped, of course; foreseeing that the hospital administrators would be absorbed into the new service, they transferred the best elsewhere in County Hall and offloaded those of lesser calibre.

LCC experience applied to the new hospital services

Now, in what were to be his last few years, my uncle blossomed in forging the Lewisham Hospital group into a committed and well organised service to its large catchment area. A good physician and teacher, he achieved this by wise understanding, careful planning, firm but gentle leadership, and above all by personal example. When he suddenly died the hospital all but closed as almost all the staff silently lined his funeral route.

What was his contribution to the NHS? Firstly, he remained a practising physician with a full share of beds, taking part, for instance, in early clinical trials of cortisone with Allott, the group pathologist. Thus he led by example. The new unstructured junior staff – a system inappropriately adopted from the teaching hospital model – were not, in his book, for exploitation; they were there to be trained and helped in their careers. Emergency admissions should not be contested by junior housemen, no patient was turned away from Lewisham, however full the wards, without his personal agreement, whatever the hour. The arrogance that I saw in some consultants as they flexed their professional muscles against each other, and against the common enemy – the administrators – was not for him.

Lewisham Hospital is sited in a busy area for trauma and the orthopaedic waiting list for "cold" cases grew. My uncle talked to his fellow physicians and to the surgeons; they agreed a scheme in summer months whereby a commitment to take four cold cases every week would be supported by making medical beds available to maintain the flow. In one summer the waiting list was halved and it was all done by informal friendliness. By contrast, when I qualified I worked in another hospital where the surgeons and anaesthetists outvoted the physicians. The surgical wards were immaculately equipped, but in the medical wards I had to tie a broom handle to the bed and screw a cup hook in to it in order to give a patient a blood transfusion.

Alice in Wonderland finances

In the NHS's early years there was a rigid demarcation between capital and revenue expenditure. It was an Alice in Wonderland financial system: the engineer at Lewisham showed how he could save thousands in fuel bills if he converted from coal to oil, at a cost that would be recovered in a year. But that would require capital expenditure, so could not be authorised for at least five years. The other problem was the familiar one of the Treasury's clawback of any underspend at the end of each financial year. At every hospital where I worked there would be sudden flurries of March expenditure, some of which was quite bizarre. My uncle developed his own response to panic calls from regional HQ: "We must spend £5 million by the end of March, can you help?". The next time round, he was ready. He foresaw the need for a modern outpatient block, cleared a bombed site for it and had plans drawn up. Came the next panic call and a detailed submission was immediate and successful. A new building was authorised, capable of expansion as need arose. He studied the system as you would a disease process.

On my last visit to his office my uncle showed me a paper from Oxford about organisation of services in the event of a major incident. He liked its approach. He knew about responding to wartime emergencies. Conscious of Lewisham's busy roads and complex of railways, he talked to his colleagues and to his ally, Matron Bell. Strategies were agreed. He died shortly before the great train disaster at Lewisham. Matron was rightly praised for her splendid leadership in coordinating the hospital's response. She knew what to do, of course.

The health service has made enormous technical strides since those days, but within the hospital service two areas have never been satisfactory. The wrong model was used for medical staffing in the NHS, which has never been a "service" as my uncle knew it in the LCC. Comradeship, loyalty, common purpose are harder to achieve when most of the doctors are, in effect, casual labour. More importantly, the expansion of specialist services into a blanket consultant provision, with all consultants being equal, led too often to factional rivalry and to arrogant conflict with administrators. This had a destructive effect on the traditions of commitment, service, the primacy of patient care, which epitomised my uncle's career. I believe this to have been a factor in the diminution in consultants' standing.

My uncle's authority, of course, came from within.

13: Resources and rationing in the NHS

Chris Ham

My involvement with the NHS began in 1975 when I was appointed by the University of Leeds to write the history of the Leeds Regional Hospital Board. Searching through the archives, interviewing those who were responsible for setting up the NHS, and analysing the literature made me realise that NHS funding has been an issue of contention since the service's inception. The estimates of likely expenditure on the NHS, made by the founding fathers, were too low and the Treasury had to find additional resources as early as 1948 to fill the gap. The imposition of an expenditure ceiling quickly followed, as did controls over manpower. More controversially, the Attlee government introduced charges for prescriptions, dental care, and spectacles, prompting the resignation from the Labour government of Nye Bevan and Harold Wilson.

These events foreshadowed later developments and bear an uncanny resemblance to the position in 1997, when one of the first acts of the new Labour government was to reiterate its commitment to control public expenditure tightly and further to reduce management costs. At the time of writing the government has not proposed to introduce new charges for treatment though this has not been ruled out as part of the comprehensive review of public spending initiated by the Treasury. To this extent, the wheel has turned full circle or, more accurately, has completed another cycle in an established pattern of policy development.

Whether the NHS is committed to repeat past behaviours or is able to break out into a different kind of future is the central question facing health policy analysts. While the inertia of such a large institution points to continuity, the pressures under which the NHS is operating may force a radical response. Paradoxically, it might be easier for the political party that created the NHS to contemplate far reaching alternatives than its Conservative opponent. Indeed, at a time when Prime Minister Tony Blair is leaving no stone unturned in his mission thoroughly to modernise the Labour Party, it would be surprising if the NHS were to escape his attentions.

Some lessons of the past

In considering options for the future, I will rehearse some lessons of the past. The first major inquiry into the cost of the NHS, the Guillebaud Report, was completed in 1956. It concluded that overall the NHS was performing well, with little evidence of extravagance or waste. Drawing on an analysis carried out by Brian Abel-Smith and Richard Titmuss, the Guillebaud Committee argued that, if anything, the NHS was underfunded and required an injection of both capital and revenue funds. In giving the NHS a clean bill of health, the committee was not oblivious to the scope for using existing resources more wisely but it laid to rest (at least temporarily) the claim of some critics that socialised medicine was inherently expensive and inefficient.

Later analyses reached similar conclusions. The report of the Royal Commission on the NHS was published in 1979, chaired by Sir Alec Merrison, it made many suggestions for improving the organisation and delivery of health care but saw no reason to move away from a health service funded through taxation and available to all on the basis of need. More surprisingly, this was also the conclusion of the reviews carried out in the 1980s under Prime Minister Margaret Thatcher. As the memoirs of Mrs Thatcher's cabinet colleagues testify, radical alternatives were considered but rejected on the basis that the methods of financing and delivery found outside the UK exhibited even more weaknesses than the NHS and that a switch from tax funding to private insurance or other alternatives would be to leap from the frying pan into the fire. Though amounting to less than a ringing endorsement of the NHS model, this nevertheless helps to explain the caution of the Conservative Government in its approach to reform. That government may have been radical in the changes it introduced to the organisation and provision of health care but it was not willing to alter fundamentally the way in which resources were raised through taxation.

Long term funding pressures remain

One of the consequences is that the long term funding pressures confronting the NHS remain. To be sure, the NHS was able to develop its services in the early 1990s but this was associated with a period in which the level of resources made available by the government was higher than in earlier years. The generosity of the Treasury ended in 1994 and by 1996 the pressures which forced Margaret Thatcher to initiate her 1988 review of the NHS had reappeared. With hospitals obliged to use trolleys to care for patients admitted as emergencies and with waiting list cases cancelled to enable priority to be given to emergency care, the NHS came to resemble a piece of elastic stretched to its limits, with no slack available to deal with new demands. With mental health services in the spotlight following well publicised cases of failures in care, both by the NHS and the local

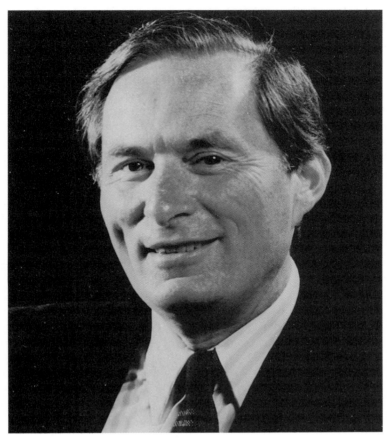

Sir Alec Merrison, former Vice Chancellor of Bristol University. He chaired the Royal Commission set up by Harold Wilson in 1976 to review the NHS. The commission reported in 1979 just after Margaret Thatcher had succeeded Wilson at the start of 18 years of Conservative rule. Reproduced with permission from Bristol University Archive.

authorities, there was hardly an area of service provision which appeared to be moving forward positively. Even general practice, elevated to the centre of the policy agenda through the initiative on a primary care-led NHS, faced staffing and recruitment difficulties as general practitioners drew attention to rising demands and declining morale.

Yet before concluding that the NHS is on its death bed, it is as well to remember the observation by a former Tory Minister of Health, Enoch Powell, that:

> One of the most striking features of the National Health Service is the continual, deafening chorus of complaint which rises day and night from every part of it, a chorus only interrupted when someone suggests that a different system altogether might be preferable, which would involve the money coming from some less (literally) palpable source. The universal Exchequer financing of the service endows everyone providing as well as using it with a vested interest in denigrating it, so that it presents what must be a unique spectacle of an undertaking that is run down by everyone engaged in it.

Like the boy who cried wolf, the risk for NHS staff and the organisations which represent their interests is that by highlighting the shortcomings of the NHS they will make it more difficult for a real crisis to be recognised when it arrives. This point is underlined by the work of analysts who conclude that there is little hard evidence that the NHS is under greater pressure than in the past. Indeed, some economists and public health specialists go further and maintain that there is considerable scope for using resources more efficiently. In particular, they argue that many medical interventions have not been properly evaluated and more could be done by increasing efficiency within the NHS and by channelling resources into areas where they will achieve most benefit for patients. These arguments are an important reminder that there is little consensus on the adequacy of NHS funding and that the level of resources required to provide a comprehensive and universal health service is an inherently contested issue.

We should remember that the UK is not alone in considering whether it can continue to provide services to the whole population from the cradle to the grave. Countries with quite different levels of health care expenditure are arguing about resources and rationing and, in the process, are testing out a range of approaches. These encompass defining core services to be funded under Medicaid in Oregon, developing service guidelines and priority criteria for waiting lists in New Zealand, and articulating an ethical platform to inform decision making in Sweden. Of particular interest is the approach adopted in The Netherlands, where a series of criteria have been identified for determining whether a service should be included in the health benefits package and where clinicians and patients are brought into the attempt to ensure that resources are used on services of proven effectiveness.

The international interest in setting priorities reflects the universal challenge of meeting all health care needs in circumstances in which resources are tightly constrained. This challenge becomes even greater at a time when politicians and the public seem to oppose an increase in taxation as a way of raising more resources for public expenditure on health care. So, unsurprisingly, radical options for reform are once again up for discussion.

Menu of options

To return to the UK, politicians prepared to think the unthinkable have a menu of options. One relatively modest but still controversial possibility would be to increase user charges, limit exemptions to existing charges, and introduce new charges, for example, for consulting a GP or staying in hospital. A second option would be to reduce the scope of the NHS by defining and limiting the list of services it provides, Oregon style. A further, much more radical, possibility would be to target the NHS on groups in the population most in need, such as people who are unemployed and on low incomes, leaving the rest to take out private medical insurance.

Each of these alternatives has drawbacks. Increasing and extending charges might raise some additional resources and deter inappropriate use but they would be costly to collect and could act as a deterrent to those groups who most need quick access to necessary medical care. A theoretical possibility is to define the core services to be funded by the NHS, but other countries which have chosen this path have encountered significant difficulties along the way. Even greater objections can be raised to targeting the NHS on part of the population only. The United States is the one developed country that has opted for this approach and its record in inequity, barriers to access, and increases in costs serves as a cautionary tale for reformers contemplating this option.

My own judgement on future funding options, reflecting on UK and international experiences, is summarised in the box.

In this context, two issues arise. Firstly, what are the respective merits of different forms of public funding? The UK has become accustomed to funding its health services via taxes raised nationally, but there are alternatives. These include local taxes, earmarked (hypothecated) taxes, and National Insurance contributions which are a tax in all but name. At a time of resistance to taxes in general, earmarked taxes or a revised form of National Insurance contributions are worth exploring as ways of supplementing the resources raised in other ways. Not least, the apparent

---

On future funding options I see ...

- no alternative to public finance as the main way of paying for health care, if basic social goals such as access, equity and comprehensiveness are important;
- public finance taking the form of taxation or social insurance or a mixture of these two;
- private finance being a valuable supplement to public finance;
- the real debate for the future being less to do with the superiority of public or private funding than how the two might best be combined to ensure adequate resources for health care.

---

willingness of the majority of the public to pay more in taxes if they know the revenue will be spent on specific services like health care suggests that these merit further consideration. This is especially important in relation to long term care, where much of the evidence points in the direction of compulsory social insurance as the most effective way of bridging the funding gap. To be sure, there are disadvantages in the social insurance option, including the effects on industrial competitiveness under a system in which both employees and employers contribute to the insurance pool, but these disadvantages seem to be less serious than those which arise in relation to other funding possibilities.

Private funding

The second issue concerns how private funding can contribute a higher proportion of total health expenditure in the future. Providing tax relief to encourage more people to take out private medical insurance is one possibility but seems to have been ruled out by the Labour Government's desire to remove this legacy of Thatcherism. Another option is to allow more discretionary spending within the NHS. This idea is favoured by some analysts because it would be a way of raising additional funds and of securing the commitment of all groups to the NHS rather than encouraging people's exit to the private sector. Examples could include extra amenities during hospital treatment and access to services that are not currently available, such as acupuncture. Providers might also levy charges if users requested a particular drug which doctors determined was therapeutically similar to an alternative but was more expensive or to provide services demanded by patients in circumstances in which there was no clinical reason for them. In this way, public and private finance could contribute together to the funding of an adequate level of services. Similarly, if compulsory social insurance is introduced to pay for long term care, this could be used to fund a basic level of provision, with clients given discretion to spend more than this to obtain additional benefits.

The NHS's 50th anniversary is an opportunity for open debate on these and other options. For too long, politicians have been "in denial" on the question of health service funding and the Labour Government's recognition that a problem exists is the first step towards a solution. The balance between public and private funding is, of course, ultimately a matter of social and political choice, reflecting the values which shape decisions on taxation and spending. The kind of health service that will be provided in the next millennium hinges on the outcome of this choice.

14:   The BMA and the NHS

John Havard

What has been the most significant achievement of the BMA in its dealings with the NHS? I believe it is the way it has managed to keep a fiercely independent profession together for half a century while negotiating its terms and conditions of service with a monopoly employer. Allied to this has been its success in pioneering the concept of a highly effective professional union while remaining implacably opposed to the more unacceptable features of industrial unionism, such as the closed shop.

For the NHS's first 25 years there was always the threat of a split between general practitioners (GPs) and consultants, mainly over differentials in remuneration and career earnings. The BMA's General Medical Services Committee (GMSC), which represents NHS GPs and acts as the executive of the Conference of Local Medical Committees, had amassed extensive experience in collective bargaining under the pre-NHS National Health Insurance Acts. When necessary the GMSC was able to arm its negotiators with the undated resignations of GPs, backed up by a large trust fund. This had been accumulated since 1919 for the purpose of providing compensation if the resignations from the state scheme ever had to be submitted. It is a tribute to the skill of their negotiators that they never were submitted.

When the government set up the collective bargaining machinery of Whitley Councils to deal with the terms and conditions of service of NHS staff, it was intended that the GMSC should act as the staff side representing GPs. The GMSC would have none of it, however, and insisted from the start on negotiating directly with the Ministry of Health. On the face of it, the Joint Consultants Committee (JCC), which formed the staff side for NHS consultants and specialists, was not so well placed. The JCC consisted of one representative from each of the six royal colleges and six from the BMA's Consultants and Specialists Committee and it eventually had to withdraw altogether from the negotiations when the colleges discovered that their charitable status, to which valuable tax concessions were attached, was in danger. The BMA committee then assumed sole negotiating responsibility.

The GP/consultant pay differential

The early days of the NHS saw mounting dissatisfaction among GPs over the differentials in remuneration and career earnings, which at that time greatly favoured consultants, despite the consultants' relatively weak negotiating position. Matters came to a head with the independent review body's first pay award in 1962. Arrangements for GPs' remuneration were based on a "pool" into which the government paid a fixed sum of money (uprated from time to time) for every GP principal in the NHS. The pool was then distributed as gross income to GPs – namely, pay plus expenses, the latter based on the average of all GPs' expenses – mainly in the form of capitation fees. The sanctity of this arrangement had become an article of belief in BMA House for many years – too many in my view – because of the security it was thought to offer against the possibility of a future glut of GPs. Furthermore, the memory of the Danckwerts arbitration of 1952,* which had effectively doubled the amount paid by the government into the GPs' remuneration pool, remained fresh in everyone's mind.

The snag was that monies earned by GPs from other official sources (for example, for services to government departments, hospitals or local health authorities) had to be deducted from the pool before it was distributed to them in the form of increased capitation fees. Unfortunately, an exceptionally large deduction had to be made in 1963, in part owing to the very large number of polio inoculations for which they had been paid the previous year. As a result the increase in net income was far less than the 14% that had been recommended by the review body.

There followed throughout the country the angriest meetings of doctors I have ever attended. Though in its next award the review body agreed that earnings from official sources (other than the NHS) should no longer be deducted, the award was less than a third of what had been claimed by the profession. Furthermore, most of it was earmarked by the review body for various schemes, including the introduction of distinction awards, anathema to GPs.

This award added fuel to the fire and the Family Doctors' Charter was hastily compiled and submitted to the ministry for negotiation, backed up by GPs' undated resignations held at BMA House. The resulting new contract led to dramatic improvements in the conditions of NHS practice for GPs. But the review body was on unfamiliar ground in having to price an entirely new contract and the eventual outcome of its next award was an increase averaging 33·3% for GPs as compared with only 10% for consultants. This almost reversed a differential that had previously greatly favoured consultants. Needless to say, a start was made on drafting a charter for consultants but the Ministry, not surprisingly, was less than

---

(* See chronology of NHS, p181)

enthusiastic and it took until 1980 to obtain significant improvements in consultants' contracts that reflected their increasing workload and responsibilities.

Constitutional changes

In the NHS's early days, the presence of non-members on the two BMA committees negotiating on behalf of NHS GPs and consultants was highly contentious, as was their quasi-autonomous status – a pragmatic BMA compromise (see below) – which the BMA's representative meeting in 1950 decided would have to be renewed annually thereafter. The questions of autonomy came to a head in 1972 with publication of the controversial report on the BMA's constitution commissioned from Sir Paul Chambers, an ex-chairman of ICI and the architect of the PAYE system of taxation. He recommended abolition of the autonomy enjoyed by both committees and the removal of non-members from all BMA committees. To an outsider it may have been a logical solution to streamline the BMA's complex representative structure and restrict committee membership to those doctors who paid their subscription to belong to the association. But his plan split the representative meeting right down the middle. Though the meeting voted to accept the Chambers Report "in its entirety" by 153 votes to 149, this vote failed to achieve the two thirds majority required for constitutional change. But the risk of the two committees splitting off from the BMA had now become more than a possibility and the minds of medicopolitical activists were sharply focused on the possible consequences. A split profession would be a dangerously weakened one.

At a further meeting the following year, Sir Paul's main recommendations were rejected. Representatives resolved that both the autonomy of the two committees and the position on them of non-members be reaffirmed and that the same should apply to "any other committee of comparable stature", adding as an example the Hospital Junior Staffs Group Council, which was not at that time even a standing committee of the BMA. The depth of feeling at the meeting was such that a roll call was demanded, each member being required to stand up when named to vote. Sir Paul had spent two years producing his report, but had failed to interview several senior members of the BMA staff, including the author, who was at that time Secretary of one of the two committees concerned. They could have advised him of the practical advantages of craft autonomy under the BMA's umbrella.

The decision was crucial to the BMA's future role in negotiating terms and conditions of the profession in the NHS. It enabled BMA committees, provided they did nothing adversely affecting another committee's interests, to negotiate their own terms and conditions of service without involving the BMA Council or the Representative Body. The new arrangement was beneficial not only for individual members, who felt their own interests were better served, but also for the BMA's representative meetings which, after consequential constitutional changes had taken place, no longer had to suffer long and tedious debates on complex issues affecting terms and conditions of service which did not apply to them. The representative meetings became far more interesting with more time being given to issues of general importance to the profession, the NHS, and the health of the community. The BMA's reputation was enhanced accordingly. Another significant outcome was to improve the status of junior doctors within the BMA. They had come close to breaking away from the GP/consultant dominated association in the late 1960s: this change gave them a stronger voice, which they used with effect.

Trade union as well as professional association

The BMA had always recognised that collective action might have to be taken against the monopoly NHS employer and that doctors would have to receive some compensation against the ensuing loss of income. However, a proviso to the BMA's Memorandum of Association prevented it from becoming a trade union, as did its status as a company limited by guarantee.

Furthermore, even if it became a trade union, it could not claim immunity from prosecution by its NHS monopoly employers for inducing

---

BMA "never knew when it had won"

Long before the NHS arrived, a political sage observed that the trouble with the BMA was that it never knew when it had won. Sometimes it does not know when it cannot win. Occasionally, much effort has been wasted on hopeless causes such as total opposition to the introduction of a limited list of NHS drugs and to any restrictions on the use of deputising services when early compromise could well have achieved better results and done less damage to the BMA's reputation.

On the other hand, the BMA's well organised and determined opposition to the introduction of NHS trusts and the market model of health care, while unsuccessful, persuaded the majority of Tory voters against them and has placed the BMA in good standing with the new administration.

Whatever may be in store for the NHS in the future, the BMA is well placed to protect the interests of doctors in the NHS as well as of patients – notwithstanding their translation into clients, consumers or, worse still, customers. Rarely do governments act on health issues without consulting the BMA as the voice of the profession. The association will, I believe, continue to have this national standing.

---

breaches of contract because doctors were not regarded as "workers" under the existing legislation. The BMA ingeniously circumvented these obstacles. It set up a Guild in 1950, administered by trustees, which could do things that the BMA was not allowed to do. In effect, the Council or any of its committees, whenever intent on taking such action, would adjourn and reconstitute itself for the purpose as a committee of the Guild. Once the necessary action had been taken to achieve a negotiating objective, it would reconvene as a BMA committee.

It seems extraordinary now that the BMA got away with this arrangement for so long. Though it was partly able to circumvent the Industrial Relations Act of 1971 by a further ruse, there was no way round trade union legislation introduced three years later and the BMA had to decide whether to register as a trade union (the new law now included doctors as workers) or to stop negotiating the terms and conditions of services of the medical profession in the NHS. The Representative Body in 1975 voted to delete the proviso in the Memorandum of Association and the BMA promptly registered as a trade union. One consequence of this, which attracted little notice, was that the BMA had to relinquish the patronage of H.M. The Queen.

1975 could hardly have been a more propitious year for the BMA to have become a trade union. That year "industrial" action took place on three fronts. Reacting to Barbara Castle's determination to stop private practice in NHS hospitals, consultants were treating only emergencies and other urgent cases while, of course, continuing to care for patients already under their care. Junior hospital doctors were restricting their work to a 40 hour week as a consequence of the slow progress being made in negotiations on their new contract and undated resignations were being collected from GPs against the probability of the government refusing to accept a review body pay award.

Industrial relations service for members

The BMA soon took advantage of its new status by launching an industrial relations service for members. This was a courageous decision as the cost was substantial and the BMA was only just emerging from a serious financial crisis. Industrial relations officers (IROs) were appointed and given a rigorous training programme. In most instances they proved to be more than a match for health service management. Objections from GPs that the new and expensive service would benefit only salaried NHS doctors were soon dropped when it was revealed that the IROs were actually spending more time helping GPs over disputes with their own staff than helping hospital doctors. The service is undoubtedly one of the main reasons why membership of the BMA has doubled over the past 20 years.

It has proved indispensable to members with the introduction of trusts and the market model of health care.

BMA's complex relations with the NHS

To do justice to the BMA's complex relations with the NHS, I would need 10,000 rather than 2000 words. For example, there were its reactions to successive NHS reorganisations, royal commissions, and other reports; its attitude to the long drawn out problems of hospital medical staffing; its attempts to obtain NHS drugs for private patients; its representation of public health doctors, junior hospital doctors, and academic staff working in the NHS; its fight against the recent health service reforms; the continuing saga of underfinancing of the service; and the BMA's many reports on health and social issues that help to inform public debate.

Over the past 50 years, the BMA has staunchly defended the profession's clinical independence and successfully represented its members' interests while respecting those of patients. With the NHS rarely out of the headlines, the BMA has also effectively ensured that the press, politicians and public know doctors' views on the service's many and diverse activities and this has influenced the policy makers.

15: Medical education and the NHS: a symbiosis

Jack Howell

The NHS began during my clinical years but I cannot recall it making a significant difference to our way of life as students. Few if any of us realised how rapidly our world was changing, both in medical knowledge and in the organisation of the health services. Our main academic task was to study the structure and functions of the human body in health and disease. Fifty years ago our knowledge was more limited than that of today's students. In the 19th century such knowledge was even scantier. Then few effective therapeutic agents were available and doctors' ability to influence the natural history of most disease was small. Medical education was dominated by the art of diagnosis and caring for sick individuals, skills achieved largely by apprenticeship to apothecaries and experienced clinicians.

As our understanding of anatomy, physiology, pharmacology, and pathology increased, these subjects occupied a larger part of the curriculum. From the early part of this century, the education of a doctor became effectively divided into two phases: a largely didactic, university based preclinical phase of 2–3 years followed by a hospital based clinical phase of three years which retained a largely apprenticeship approach. The former was intended to provide the scientific basis of the medical practice but in reality this link was rarely achieved, most clinicians relying more upon pattern recognition and clinical experience.

Safe doctors

The advent of the NHS did little immediately to alter the goal of undergraduate medical education which since the Medical Act of 1886 had remained to produce a safe doctor, competent to enter general practice. He or she was expected to recognise and manage the limited range of important conditions. These included infectious diseases and remediable conditions such as anaemia, diabetes, thyrotoxicosis, and myxoedema, for which failure to recognise and treat effectively could be disastrous.

Midwifery was also commonly a part of general practice. Apart from surgery, there was little else that a doctor could do to influence the natural history of an illness and surgery of any magnitude required, though not legally, further training and experience.

The safe doctor was, for a while, an achievable goal, but in the decade before the NHS began, medical knowledge and technology began to expand dramatically, introducing means of earlier diagnosis and effective therapy and also the potential to harm as well as benefit. The inadequacy of undergraduate education to meet the broadening needs of medicine was recognised in 1944 by the Goodenough Committee, which recommended a year of clinical experience after "qualifying" before registration with the General Medical Council (GMC). But this requirement was not introduced until 1953.

The NHS Act of 1946 required the Minister of Health to promote the development of a free, comprehensive health service for all, to include prevention, treatment, and rehabilitation and in July 1948, this great social experiment began. The advent of the NHS in itself did not change the nature of medical practice, only access to it. Free access to GP services and, through them, to hospital and community care created a need for many more doctors, educated and trained to work in the new service.

Initially, the large pool of experienced doctors who had served in the armed forces easily met the needs of the new NHS. Indeed, in 1957 the Willink Committee, set up by the Department of Health, recommended a temporary reduction in medical schools' intake to avoid a predicted surplus of doctors. However, by 1964 only 1500 students a year (compared with an estimated annual need of 2500) completed their training. Along with concerns about the appropriateness of the medical curriculum for practice in the NHS, this led in 1965 to the Royal Commission on Medical Education. Chaired by Lord Todd, a Nobel prize winner in chemistry and head of a Cambridge college, the commission's report in 1968 was to have an immediate, profound, and lasting effect on medical education.

Royal Commission on Medical Education

In an interim report, the Royal Commission recognised the urgent need for more doctors because of a predicted shortfall of some 11,000 doctors in the UK by 1975. It recommended an immediate increase in the intake of medical schools and the establishment of three new medical schools, the first to be created in the United Kingdom this century. The commission's members realised that their final recommendations would "be of little value unless they provide a basis for the adequate satisfaction of the country's need, not for the immediate future, but two generations hence". So they looked forward to the likely future pattern of medical care in the NHS and produced a pattern of medical education to provide for it.

The final report presented an alternative vision of how doctors in the NHS might share professional responsibilities, a vision that called for radical changes in undergraduate and postgraduate medical education. Predicting that all doctors would be specialists in some aspects of medical care, the authors anticipated that consultants and general practitioners would be equally regarded and fully trained. Significantly, they noted that the "retention of the obsolete concept of undergraduate medical education" had been influenced by the absence of adequate arrangements for postgraduate professional training.

Emphasising that the university education of a doctor must incorporate practical instruction, the Royal Commission concluded that this could be given only as a part of "the provision of medical care through the health services of the nation", an explicit recognition of the symbiotic relationship of the NHS and medical education. The report envisaged the aim of undergraduate medical education not as the production of a "finished" doctor but of "a broadly educated man (*sic*) who can become a doctor by further training". This emphasis on the need for continuing education of all doctors accelerated the development of postgraduate education. A further 30 years has passed, however, before we have reached the current position, where each NHS region has an established postgraduate structure with its own budget, recently strengthened by the appointment of directors of medical education in the major health service trusts.

Undergraduate medical education

What of the recommendations for producing a "broadly educated man" by which the Royal Commission clearly meant an individual who had knowledge not only of the "facts" of the traditional subjects of anatomy, physiology, biochemistry, pathology, etc. but also those additional subjects which had become important in the NHS. Among these were sociology and human relationships, the psychology of individuals and families, community medicine and public health, clinical epidemiology, statistics, and the use of computers. Like the GMC, the Royal Commission emphasised the need to control the increasing amount of detail taught in each discipline and specialty and to ensure that the student had time and opportunity to study the principles on which medicine is based.

The establishment of academic clinical units in all medical schools, as recommended in the Goodenough Report, ensured that the scientific basis of medicine could be taught, often jointly with preclinical departments, but there were many difficulties in offering a balanced and relevant clinical experience. For example, as Sir Francis Walshe observed in 1971, patients admitted to teaching hospitals tended to be selected, favouring the rare or the difficult illnesses; furthermore, the nature of the training of the teaching hospital consultant tended to lead to a dominantly vocational approach to the education of students.

Changing the curriculum: Southampton's model

In recommending changes, the Royal Commission was not prescriptive; it endorsed the GMC's recommendations that each university should be free to develop its own ideas with as little restriction as possible. All medical schools were urged to revise their curricula, but radical change to an existing curriculum is difficult and the new schools were at an advantage. They had freedom to design their own curriculum from scratch, subject to inspection and approval by the GMC. Each new school sought to make medical education more relevant by incorporating the main Royal Commission recommendations in their own individual way. I have personal knowledge only of the curriculum at the medical school at Southampton University, one of the three post–Todd schools.

To capitalise on the enthusiasm with which students entered medical school, throughout the first year the medical school arranged for them to visit patients with a variety of chronic illnesses in their home. They would then learn early on what it meant to an individual and the family to be ill. Fortunately, communication was rarely a problem at this early stage, though too often it tended to become so as students and young doctors progressed through their careers.

The new curriculum included behavioural and social sciences, community medicine, clinical epidemiology, statistics, ethics and even management. We also made radical changes to the overall structure which blurred the traditional distinction between preclinical and clinical phases. The school replaced anatomy and physiology with "systems courses" where the anatomy, physiology, pharmacology, pathology, and mechanisms of disease of each system were presented together and illustrated by clinical demonstrations. The absence of individual disciplines had disadvantages, but the horizontal integration between systems allows students' understanding of the abnormal to illuminate the normal. They could develop robust models of the body in health and disease and so, the teaching staff hoped, establish a better basis for the clinical experience that would follow. This approach was a success and the GMC now explicitly recommends such systems courses. A logical consequence was to replace the traditional second MB examination in preclinical subjects with a broader, even more rigorous examination, which included mechanisms of disease, at the end of the third year when students had had the opportunity to develop clinical skills and to "clerk" patients.

Perhaps the most radical change we faced was how to interpret what the Royal Commission considered essential for an "educated man". Our solution was to require the student to undertake a substantial research project for most of the fourth year, not only to appreciate the nature of knowledge by attempting to add to it themselves but also so that current practice should be constantly tested and developed as knowledge generally advances. That distinguished Regius Professor of Medicine at Oxford, Sir George Pickering, described this year as the only worthwhile experiment in medical education that had taken place in his lifetime.

Congested teaching hospitals prompt switch to regional hospitals

The new schools had a further advantage: they were not associated with established teaching hospitals. In July 1948, voluntary and municipal hospitals were placed under the control of one of the 14 regional hospital boards (RHBs), except for the teaching hospitals, which had their own board of governors accountable directly to the Minister of Health. These hospitals were separately and more generously funded to take account of their teaching and research roles and their positions as centres of clinical excellence. The consequence was that they became somewhat isolated and insulated from the rest of the NHS. An unfortunate outcome of this isolation was the concentration of clinical teaching in these hospitals: this created congestion in the wards and outpatient departments as the students of three clinical years sought hands-on experience.

Yet, apart from some *ad hoc* arrangements with individual consultants, a great teaching resource lay virtually unused in neighbouring RHB hospitals: there students could get greater clinical experience and personal supervision. Because the new medical schools were developed in co-operation with the RHB, they had easier access to the region's hospitals.

A most formidable challenge

- Given the rapid rate of changes in health care, the GMC guidance of 1993 will be invaluable for medical schools, which need to produce roundly educated and professionally adaptable doctors.
- In addition to the ever increasing advances in medical knowledge and technology, the responsibilities of doctors themselves are changing. Limited resources no longer allow doctors in the NHS to act solely in the interest of individual patients, as enshrined in the Hippocratic Oath: the need to prioritise care in the interests of all patients may conflict with the doctor's primary ethical responsibility to the individual patient.
- I see this as one of the profession's most formidable challenges and urge the NHS and the medical schools to ensure that the education of students and doctors prepares them for their role in tomorrow's NHS.

At Southampton medical school, for example, we invited every district general hospital (DGH) in the Wessex region to take clinical students as apprentices in their final year and all accepted. This meant that rather than several students per firm, often from each of three years, there would be only
one final year student with the opportunity to be a "shadow houseman" and gain considerable supervised experience and encouragement to study. At the end of the attachment, students are examined jointly by the consultant and a visiting clinical academic, with the result contributing to his or her final examination results. This arrangement has been running for more than 20 years and I can testify that the initial fears of some senior doctors over standards of quality have proved ill founded. Not until the NHS reorganisation of 1974 were boards of governors abolished, with teaching hospitals becoming accountable to the RHB. Since then the use of DGHs for teaching students has spread nationwide, though cuts in the numbers of beds and a higher turnover of patients is putting this teaching resource under strain (p153.). Teaching by GPs in their surgeries has also provided wider clinical experience as part of students' first clinical attachments in their third year.

The older established medical schools also began to change but more slowly and with greater difficulty. In 1979, the Royal Commission on the NHS, chaired by Sir Alec Merrison, noted criticism that the medical curriculum "was inappropriate to the need of the NHS". Though recognising the occurrence of some changes in the direction recommended by the Todd Report, Merrison commented that these were "not enough". He and his fellow commissioners looked to the newly reconstituted GMC (1978) to use its new powers to do more. The GMC's *Recommendations on Undergraduate Medical Education* (published in 1993) and *The New Doctor* (1997), directed at the preregistration year, outline the essentials of a curriculum and clinical training better able to prepare young doctors for their continuing long term education in the NHS or elsewhere.

16: Reflections on quality in general practice

Sir Donald Irvine

I was at school when the NHS began. My family lived in the Northumberland coal mining community of Ashington, where my father was in singlehanded general practice. Life for mining families was tough. Miners were in a physically demanding and dangerous occupation which resulted in high morbidity and mortality. For most women, maintaining the family in often difficult home and economic conditions was still their life, though many younger women had tasted independence through wartime factory work.

General practice was an integral part of our family life. Consultations were at the house. I remember "going on visits" at weekends and in holidays; the huge, straw-wrapped glass "carboys" of medicines which we all helped to unpack; the immaculate white wrapping paper, fixed with red sealing wax for every bottle of medicine; and the regular sound of my father going out at night – almost every night – to attend a "confinement" or medical emergency.

The new NHS brought mixed feelings in our household. There was hope that it would improve care by making specialists more accessible and remove worries for many about the cost of care to ill people. But there was also caution. For GPs, the future in the NHS seemed far from certain. The "free" service unleashed a pent-up demand for care which overwhelmed many doctors. Furthermore, general practitioners were seen as dropouts from mainstream medicine by the rapidly expanding, confident and assertive specialties, as I found as a medical student.

As if to drive the point home, Joseph Collings, a New Zealand trained GP reporting at that time on the fitness of GPs to play an effective part in the new NHS, published a damning report on the general quality of practice. His view – shared by most specialists – was that, unless radically changed, general practice was incapable of rising to the responsibilities for primary care and prevention envisaged in the new NHS.

GPs responded angrily. The most important constructive reaction came from those determined practitioners who, like my father, followed the lead of the late John Hunt to join in founding the College of General Practitioners (now with a royal prefix) in 1952. Acknowledging reality, in particular the apparently huge variation in quality, they thought that the college should set general standards of practice and education, so that the future would not depend totally on the motivation, sense of responsibility, and whim of individual doctors.

Early experience of the NHS

After graduation and two years of house jobs, I joined my father for what was to become an excellent apprenticeship – today we call it vocational training. During the next five years I gained important insights on quality which, though a reflection of the NHS as it then was, still hold good today.

First and foremost, I learnt at first hand from my father's patients just what quality of medical care meant for them. It was about very easy access to "my doctor" linked with continuity of care. They wanted a doctor whom they could trust, who would find out what was wrong with them and who would help them and their families to cope with the impact of illness on their everyday lives. Quality was, in a nutshell, about expertise, ethical behaviour, and a powerful vocational commitment to service. These were (and still are) the pillars on which good quality medical practice rested. My father was typical of many family doctors who practised in this way. Unfortunately, just as many others did not, as Collings had shown.

Secondly, I learnt about the power and value of data and information and the difficulties the absence of these posed when trying to describe practice. I saw this first in the huge frustration that outstanding family doctors like the late Andrew Smith felt when they were unable to explain coherently to sceptical specialists how and why the patterns of disease, and the presentation of illness in general practice, were so different from hospital practice and what this meant for the management of patients outside hospital. John Fry, Keith Hodgkin, and Donald Crombie made the first studies recording morbidity in general practice which, when published, confirmed a picture of ill health in the community quite different from that experienced by medical students in teaching hospitals.

Thirdly, I learnt the value of systematic peer review. In the early 1960s most seriously ill patients were still seen at home, so daily visiting lists of 20 and more were the rule. At the end of each evening surgery my father would "make up the list" by having a semi-formal discussion for about an hour. The intention was that each of us would know what was going on, could talk over questions of diagnosis and management and, where appropriate, could give a second opinion on a difficult case next day. He created a climate in which we could question each other's management without anyone taking offence. He saw this process of review as a normal and important part of everyday operational and clinical management, of "knowing your practice". Random case analysis, critical incident review, and case based audit in today's general practice have their roots in experiences such as this. Indeed, the very latest quality developments still reflect the idea of "knowing your practice" well.

Next, I recognised that the kind of apprenticeship I had experienced was highly unusual, an accident of birth and circumstance. By 1964, five years into general practice, I had learnt much about the educational value of case review, how to gather and analyse data, how to use a library, and how to write. Clinical apprenticeship and, in my case, the "higher" training inherent in doing an MD degree from general practice on a clinical subject were elements of quality in medicine taken for granted in the hospital specialties and yet wholly a matter of personal preference in general practice. For me, this early experience simply reinforced the views then being vigorously pursued by family doctors like John Hunt, John Horder, and Patrick Byrne that a basic building block for quality in NHS general practice must be vocational training for all.

Lastly, I saw that the traditional "do it all yourself" approach to the organisation of general practice could not be sustained in the face of growing pressure for more sophisticated cure and care. The way forward was being explored by pioneers like Ecke Kuensberg, George Swift and Geoffrey Marsh, who were bringing basic administrative support and organisation to their practices and experimenting with the attachment of district nurses and health visitors. They and likeminded enthusiasts, harnessing their efforts through the college, laid the practice foundations for the Family Doctors' Charter of 1964.

Improving the structure, raising the quality

Prior to the charter, the life of general practice in the NHS hung by a thread. The Charter negotiations, led so ably by James Cameron, was hailed by the BMA, rightly, as a great victory for the profession over the parsimonious instincts of the government. It was largely the result of two factors. Firstly, there was courageous pioneering in the field by a minority of general practitioners who were showing the way ahead in the face of considerable opposition to change from colleagues. Secondly, general practice was fortunate in having the influential support of the Chief Medical Officer, Sir George Godber, who did so much behind the scenes to keep the eyes of government on the potential of modern general practice. I remember him saying to me later, "it was touch and go – we nearly lost it" (p15).

The charter agreement established group practice and provided a secure basis for improving its structure – the buildings, equipment, staffing, records and so on. Much of general practice has since been modernised, with purpose built premises and the evolution of the primary care team. So, though there are still significant gaps, particularly in some inner city areas, the quality of the environment for primary care has improved beyond recognition.

The environment for care is important, but for patients what matters most is whether their doctors know what they are doing and whether they care. The recognition, from within general practice, that particular knowledge, skills, and attitudes were needed to provide a good personal service went to the heart of patients' agendas. Simply qualifying as a doctor, it was said, would of itself no longer suffice. So, in the late 1960s and 1970s, the profession and the NHS together made a significant effort to establish postregistration vocational training. In this, *The Future General Practitioner*, published by the RCGP in 1972, was a landmark in providing the intellectual underpinning of general practice as a specialty in its own right.

Aiming for a quality, primary care-led NHS

- The achievement of good quality care is critically dependent on sufficient investment to ensure good data describing process and outcome. Quality without data is a contradiction in terms.
- This is all the more remarkable because the NHS prides itself on technical expertise in clinical practice and has had the nation's health as well as the well-being of individual people as a basic objective.
- Now, we talk openly of a primary care-led NHS and other countries look with envy at our system of general practice which is right for modern times.
- This achievement, absolutely unthinkable when the NHS began, is a tribute to a quality-led renaissance of which all who have played their part can be justly proud.

One decision was to have a significant impact – at the time not foreseen – on the quality of general practice as a whole. The college, recognising the powerful influence of modelling in medical education, decided that young doctors should only be allowed to gain experience in specially selected "teaching" practices which could show a good standard of teaching and patient care. Thus, there were to be explicit standards for both teaching general practitioners and their practices and verification of compliance through external peer review. And accountability would be strengthened by using time limited appointments, with renewal subject to satisfactory performance. In terms of quality, much that has happened in general practice since then has, with varying degrees of success, built upon this first experience of accountability based on explicit standards, performance monitoring, and peer review.

Vocational training transformed NHS general practice, hugely improving confidence and morale. Furthermore, many observers say that the trained generations of general practitioners are much better prepared for their work than their predecessors. I am sure that is true.

Quality comes of age

The 1980s and 1990s gave a further turn to the quality wheel. At the same time, this illustrated some of the real difficulties in extending the general principles of quality from enthusiasts across the whole profession, though I like to think that the experiences of improving teaching and quality in general practice have positively influenced training and quality in the hospital based specialties.

Once again, it was the RCGP which took the next steps. Building on experience in selecting teaching practices, it introduced a more rigorous way of looking at practice performance called *What Sort of Doctor?* And, in 1983, the College launched its Quality Initiative, the object of which was to try to bring quality improvement and quality assurance to every practice within ten years. Within this, the more narrowly defined medical audit was gaining momentum among enthusiasts. But professionally led initiatives proved insufficient. It was this recognition that led the government, through the 1990 health reforms, to try itself to make all doctors, in hospitals as well as general practice, more accountable for the quality of their work. Hence the new contract for GPs, income related continuing education, the postgraduate educational allowance, the NHS clinical audit programme, the clinical effectiveness initiative, and so on.

Partnership between profession and NHS

Quality in general practice has evolved as a partnership effort between profession and NHS. Most initiatives have been professionally led by enthusiasts breaking new ground. But to secure general implementation, the government has become involved to provide the infrastructure, incentives, and contractual arrangements necessary to engage all doctors.

The biggest hole lies, paradoxically for a national health service, in a chronic inability among doctors, managers, and politicians at all levels to understand that the achievement of good quality care is critically dependent on sufficient investment to ensure good data describing process and outcome. Quality without data is a contradiction in terms. This is all the more remarkable because the NHS prides itself on technical expertise in clinical practice and has had the nation's health as well as the well-being of individual people as a basic objective. Actually, general practice is doing relatively well. Today, one is more likely to see a computer terminal on the GP's consulting room desk than in outpatients. General practice, with its population denominator in the registered list of patients and the ongoing clinical record, is well placed to exploit the coming revolution in information technology, which should help remedy this deficiency.

17: From eager immigrant to NHS consultant: an uphill trek

Abdul Jaleel

> Make it compulsory for a doctor using a brass plate to have inscribed on it, in addition to the letters indicating his qualifications, the words: "remember that I too am mortal" . (George Bernard Shaw)

Since my first day in Britain 36 years ago, little has gone to plan. I landed at Heathrow airport expecting to be met by my best friend, but he was nowhere to be seen. I drifted to the news stand where I saw with shock the evening newspaper headline announcing his death: he had been accidentally electrocuted in his home in Kensington. Fortunately for me, my friend had booked my accommodation and a course in tropical medicine at Edinburgh. I came to Britain expecting, like 95% of medical graduates from the Indian subcontinent, to return to Pakistan having completed my education. But I am still here. After Edinburgh, I accidentally fell into the National Health Service, starting a long uphill trek to the top.

As an eager young student, I inevitably compared the way a Third World health delivery system operated with the way Britain's modern, civilised health service performed. Initially, I simply noted the huge chasm between the two in terms of equity and standards of care. But as I gained my qualifications, I also recognised a great gulf in terms of job satisfaction, a persuasive factor for a young man contemplating possible careers. So eight months after arriving in this country, having obtained my qualifications in tropical medicine, I decided to make my career in a modern health service. To reach that decision was easy; to get started was more difficult. I needed a job but without experience I could not get one and without one I could not get experience: a classic Catch 22 circle.

Experience was not all I was lacking: I did not have a white skin. My peers progressed but despite making 45 applications for any and every job, I got nowhere. In the innocence of youth, I did not know how the system operated. Looking back, I believe that this was my first encounter with racial discrimination. Eventually, it was a time honoured British technique

100

which gave me a springboard into the NHS: the old boys' network. A friend in Manchester needed cover while he took a sabbatical and he asked me to step in. But that springboard could only launch me onto the lowest rung of the NHS ladder and I soon discovered that a trainee doctor was a nobody. This engaged my sense of injustice. I returned from a holiday in France in 1965 to a bill not only for occupying hospital accommodation but also for the meals that I had not eaten. I had already been outraged by a hospital matron who, ironically, hailed from Dublin. She indignantly told me that she did not approve of "her girls" hobnobbing with doctors from the colonies. Then taking me into her confidence, she explained her unhappiness with the appointment of doctors who came (even worse) from Africa. "Our patients," she declaimed, "don't want to wake up in the middle of the night to see a black figure with big white teeth wandering around".

Hospital or general practice?

As a nobody, I bit my tongue in public, did as I was told and climbed a couple of career rungs until the big decision approached: to specialise or to go into general practice. The decision was made using the same criteria which had convinced me to stay in Britain. While fashion and money beckoned me into general practice, I was still more interested in standards of care. General practice is a huge challenge, but I felt that a hospital doctor was better able to deliver a higher standard of care, albeit across a narrower spectrum of medicine. Yet discrimination resurfaced: I found it well nigh impossible to win a place in a teaching hospital and the "glamorous" specialties were, it seemed, closed to me.

Sadly, matters have not improved. In 1994 more than 20 years after my humbling experiences I read of a doctor from an ethnic minority being refused more than 1000 jobs. This did not surprise me. I pointed out in a letter to *The Times* how "uncommon [it was] to see such doctors in major teaching hospitals, large city hospitals and in the so-called glamorous medical specialties. The lucky few who climb to the top (consultant level) often end up in less popular disciplines such as geriatrics, psychiatry and genito-urinary medicine".

But by 1994 I understood why all those years before I had been unsuccessful. I had sat on many appointment committees at all levels of the NHS – often as the only member of an ethnic minority and probably with a tag saying "token" hanging around my neck – witnessing the way some applicants were weeded out. My letter in *The Times* said: "It is not uncommon to have a pecking order for short-listing, with applicants from ethnic minorities placed below the UK-born and other European Community doctors". I did, of course, question such behaviour. Nothing was said but I was never invited back.

View from the top

In 1969 I had become a Senior Registrar in rheumatology and three years later I climbed further up the NHS ladder and thought that I had just about reached the top when I became consultant at Darlington Memorial Hospital. But then I looked down ...

I came to Darlington, an historic centre of heavy engineering suffering from postindustrial decline, to establish a new department of rheumatology and rehabilitation. My predecessor was a distinguished visiting rheumatologist whose commitments elsewhere had undoubtedly affected development of his Darlington patch. On arrival I found no office, no secretary, no beds, and not even an awareness in the hospital of what a rheumatologist did! Ten years earlier when, as a junior doctor, I was confronted with the awful realisation that I was a nobody, I had managed to rein back my feelings of frustration. Now, confronted with the naked reality that my department had nothing, I was determined to put matters right. Overnight, I acquired an office and a secretary from the "nominal powers that be". Dealing with the "practical powers that were" was, however, quite different. Even in a regional hospital, bed empires, where the number of beds bearing a consultant's name were a measure of his hierarchical power, were not so easily overcome.

Rheumatology as a specialty had found its feet between the two wars but in the provinces in the early 1970s, many consultants and administrators still failed to accept or even comprehend why inpatient facilities were necessary for patients suffering from rheumatic diseases. At the time, sufferers were as often referred to unorthodox practitioners as they were to the "physical doctor". Extracting resources for a low profile service from a cash strapped regional hospital was hard work. After about six months, my senior consultant colleagues graciously allowed me eight beds on a general medical ward, though problems persisted. It took much longer to acquire junior medical staff, and when eventually they came, it was only because the consultants who had "ownership" of them wanted to do me a favour. Gradually, however, the quality of service my department could provide improved.

Challenging the power structure

Sadly, however, this specialist pecking order still exists within the health service. To many professional insiders and observers in the media and the public, heart or brain surgeons are still at the top of the tree. However, to the people who most matter – the patients for whom the NHS was designed – what is important is that their problems are treated sensitively and expeditiously by the relevant specialist. Nevertheless, by fighting my own battles I had developed a confidence to challenge the power structures that I felt were serving neither the patients nor the professionals. In 1980 I joined the local Senior Medical Staff Committee, persuaded as much by the apathy that surrounded me as by any philanthropic ambitions. Indeed, the apathy of others, perhaps inspired by their determination not to be labelled as troublemakers, pricked my conscience, prompting me to play a role, however small, in changing the power structures. I joined despite warnings from colleagues about the unwritten rule that doctors should keep out of politics. Interestingly, even when elected Secretary to the SMSC, I met with subtle racial prejudice: for example, I was not given the minute book for several weeks.

My position on the SMSC gave me a seat on the BMA's Regional Consultants Committee and the following year, I was elected to the Central Consultants Committee which represented all NHS consultants. I retired from that committee in 1997 and feel that in a small way I achieved something for my colleagues and our patients. If only more doctors were willing to contribute time and effort to medicopolitics, the profession could, I believe, greatly strengthen its influence on the course of events in the NHS. Today, health service managers at local and national levels do realise that they must consult doctors before implementing decisions which affect patient care. Doctors need to be able to give considered advice, especially as I have seen the power of consultants ebbing away during my 34 years in the NHS.

In some ways this has been a positive development because consultants had great power and not all used it constructively. For instance, when I came to Darlington, my patients were given "block bookings" for their appointments. They would just sit there in outpatients, ten or more of them, waiting for hours on end when it was patently obvious that the consultant could see only one patient at a time. When I pointed out this unsatisfactory situation to the appointments supervisor, she could not see the problem. After all, no one had complained before and this was the way appointments had been made ever since she joined the NHS in 1948. Determined consultant action could surely have made the system more patient friendly and efficient.

Society's esteem for doctors

That patients were prepared to wait interminably, though, was symbolic of the esteem in which the doctors have been held by society in general and needy patients in particular. Patients had an almost mystical belief in their doctors and their healing powers. The community still respects doctors but we must heed Bernard Shaw's reminder of our mortality. Today, better education and knowledge on the part of the patients have made them more certain of what care and standards they can expect. Regrettably, patients' rights and expectations have not always been matched by responsible behaviour on their part. And, importantly, successive governments have failed to provide resources to meet patients' needs. The increase in patient power has been accompanied by an increase in the power of managers, many of whom have become alarmingly politicised – with a small p. General practitioners, too, have increased their influence, sometimes at the expense of hospitals, and even the insurance companies are putting pressure on doctors. With the burgeoning costs of health care, our political masters and private health insurers have encroached on the regulation of patient care, previously the domain of the consultant, under the banner of "managed care". In such a climate the inevitable uncertainties of the science of medicine cannot be countenanced by management. Because the "customer" has been sold a package of care, whether tax financed or privately funded, the hospital doctor has to follow the package's predetermined path. Whatever knowledge and experience suggest is the best course for a particular patient, he or she dare not deviate from that path.

Failed revolution

The revolutionary changes sprung upon an unsuspecting nation by the politicians in 1989 were a kneejerk response to chronic underfunding of the NHS. Ironically, the changes have further highlighted the service's chronic weaknesses. The so-called internal health market – the "infernal" market as Sandy Macara, the chairman of the BMA Council, aptly termed it some years ago – has blatantly failed. A decade on, when winter comes many patients will still be unable to find beds. Market forces, so successful in the commercial sector, have singularly failed a humane, demand-led NHS. Not only have these changes demoralised staff in hospitals and the community, but they have also created anomalies. For a start, they swallowed money, which followed the bureaucrats rather than the patients, as ministers had promised. Between 1990 and 1997, the red tape needed to govern the internal market devoured an extra £1·5 billion a year. There were 20,000 more managers yet 50,000 fewer nurses. It has been easier to furnish a manager's office or to appoint extra secretarial staff for a trust director than to fill the gaps in staffing at the sharp end: in the wards or in outpatients.

I cannot write about the NHS without reference to the shift in the NHS's centre of gravity from clinical to management priorities. Let me give two personal examples which angered me since they threatened doctors' clinical independence, confidentiality of patients' medical records and confidentiality of communications between doctors. More than once, I have been asked by hospital managers for a medical report on a trust employee's fitness to work when they have quoted from my letters in the patient's medical records, presumably without permission. I have also experienced censorship by managers of consultants' correspondence with GPs, when my colleagues and I were warning that a shortage of consultants' secretaries would delay correspondence on patients. Modest breaches of accepted codes, perhaps, but also a potentially damaging trend.

The internal market has also created a two tier system of service for patients. As service providers selling a commodity, hospital doctors had to follow the bureaucratic money trail. Against my better judgement, I was forced to give preference to those patients referred by GP fundholders. The latter would receive frequent treatment sessions with the rheumatologist, whereas patients from the non-fundholding practices would be rationed to an infrequent visit to their specialist. In the silence of the waiting room, it took a while for this inequity to be unmasked. But gradually it was, and I think (indeed, I hope) that it was one reason that the electorate moved so decisively in the General Election of May 1997.

The future

- I do not believe that the United Kingdom will ape a North American style, insurance based system to provide universal health care.
- General practitioners are trained generalists with an already heavy workload. It is absurd that, as leaders of primary health care teams, they should be expected to lead the NHS. With no specialist infrastructure in the community, it would be unrealistic to expect GPs to act as minispecialists in addition to their generalist responsibilities. The cost implications are unpredictable but almost certainly large. The concept is a political gimmick that I predict will soon perish.
- Rapid advances in information technology will change the face of medical practice. Record keeping will be revolutionised and teleconsultation among doctors, between primary, secondary, and community care, and between doctors and patients will herald profound changes in the skill mix and numbers of the workforce and in working patterns. The digitalisation of diagnostic imaging will enhance the efficiency and quality of clinical services.
- Doctors should remember that they too are mortal.

The NHS is like an oceangoing liner. It will take far more than tinkering with the wheel to change its course. Meanwhile, the standards and equity of care that so impressed me all those years ago when I accidentally, and fortuitously, began my NHS career will, I fear, continue to suffer. That said, I am proud to have contributed to a service that has provided so much good care to so many people.

18: Economic and political costs of the NHS: a changing balance sheet?

Rudolf Klein

Fifty years after its birth, the NHS has taken its place among Britain's most cherished institutions. As a symbol of national pride and solidarity, it has replaced even the monarchy. Any threat to the NHS, whether real or imagined, is apt to mobilise both public and professional opinion in support of it. The political parties compete to demonstrate their dedication to it. But there is a paradox in all this. Born among conflict between politicians and the medical profession, the NHS is also a mechanism for perpetuating that conflict. Overwhelming support for the principle of the NHS goes hand in hand with endemic discontent about the way in which it functions. Crises and confrontations punctuate its history with great regularity. For governments, irrespective of party, the NHS tends to be a source of political embarrassment. For professionals working in the NHS, governments tend, again irrespective of party, to be a source of frustration and irritation.

In exploring this paradox, I start by reminding readers about what we tend to take for granted. This is that the NHS represents the institutional-isation of a vision of social justice: a collective decision that health care should be available to everyone, by right of being a resident in the UK, and that access should be solely determined by need. It is the enduring power of the ideals incorporated into the design of the NHS, buttressed by the self-interest we all have in being assured access to health care if we fall ill, which explains the continuing strong support for the NHS. But the way in which these ideals were translated into the bricks and mortar of institutional design helps to explain, in turn, the frequent sense of disappointment at its actual performance.

NHS unique

For the NHS is unique among health care systems in at least one respect. Collective, universal systems of health care provision are now the norm

106

among Western countries, the United States always excepted. But only a small group of these, notably the Scandinavian countries, have systems, like that of the United Kingdom, which are funded out of public revenues rather than insurance schemes. And even among this group, Britain stands out as the country which runs a national system financed out of taxation: where both finance and administration are centralised. In the other models, responsibility for delivering health care is generally delegated to local authorities, albeit operating within a national framework.

I do not believe that adoption of the 1948 UK model was inevitable. Most of the schemes discussed in the years leading up to 1948 had assumed a much greater degree of pluralism. If a centralised model was adopted, it was not because any other design would necessarily have failed to deliver social justice. The vision of universal access to health care could have been achieved in other ways. The centralised model was adopted because it accommodated the ambitions both of the medical profession and of the bureaucratic rationalisers in government. On the one hand, it meant that the spectre of local authority control had been exorcised: a spectre that had haunted the medical profession in the years of negotiation that preceded the creation of the NHS. On the other hand, it created an instrument which meant that resources could be distributed according to rational principles and that best medical practices could be diffused through the country.

In short, the shape that the NHS took in 1948 was at least as much a victory for doctors (though they did not recognise it as such at the time) as for Socialist idealism. It created a service in which doctors would be free to use public resources to deliver health care according to need as defined by the medical profession itself. Medical autonomy, as much as social justice, seemed to be enshrined in the design of the NHS. And here we come to the central irony: it is precisely this victory of the medical profession which explains the tensions that have characterised the NHS ever since, the sense of a utopian vision was always destined to be disappointed in practice.

Economic benefits, political costs

For governments, of whatever party, the NHS is an ambiguous blessing. Economics and politics point in opposite directions. For governments intent on keeping down public expenditure and the level of taxation (as all are, if to a lesser or greater extent), the NHS is the perfect instrument of control. The central budget, once determined, remains set in concrete: there are (the drug bill and some general practitioner activities excepted) no open-ended commitments dragging spending upward. In this respect, the NHS remains the envy of the world. It delivers reasonable quality health care to the whole population, with a reasonable degree of equity, but spending a smaller proportion of the national income on health care than most other advanced countries. If containing the health care cost explosion is the problem, as it is in many countries, then the NHS model provides the solution. I am not surprised that, despite searching the world for alternative models of financing health care, the free market Thatcher government of the 1980s in the end settled for the status quo.

But the political cost of economic success is the NHS's semipermanent crisis of "underfunding". The success story for Treasury ministers is, from the perspective of those working in the NHS, a story of inadequate resources. Successive committees of inquiry and royal commissions, from Guillebaud to Merrison as well as several non-governmental reports, have struggled to define what an adequate level of funding means and have been forced to admit defeat. Given the elasticity of the notion, ever expanding as the scope of medical intervention widens and public expectations rise, there is no firm ground on which to rest an argument. Lacking consensus about the criteria to be used in assessing the adequacy (or otherwise) of funding, the NHS has throughout its history been the stage for a debate which has varied in its bitterness over time but which remains unresolved today.

This lack of consensus explains a phenomenon first noted by Enoch Powell more than 30 years ago when reflecting on his experience as Minister of Health. Those working in the NHS, he noted, have "a vested interest in denigration". The most powerful weapon they have in the continual struggle to attract extra resources (and which profession does not think that it could deliver a better service if only it had more money?) is to advertise the shortcomings of the NHS. The language of crisis – the warnings of disaster and the shroud waving – is thus built into the design of the NHS.

From this flow the political costs of the NHS. Here I would make a simple point. The public believe doctors but not politicians. While doctors always appear at or near the top of the hierarchy of prestige (and trust) in surveys where the public are asked to rank different occupations, politicians invariably appear near the bottom. A minister spouting statistics, whether about the NHS's increased output or about a decline in patients, waiting times for hospital care, is therefore not nearly as convincing as a doctor warning that his or her patients are being put in danger because of lack of resources. In the battle of credibility, politicians are bound to be the losers.

The political costs of the NHS are further increased because of the other feature of its design that distinguishes it from health care systems elsewhere: centralisation. Centralised funding means, in turn, centralised accountability: Bevan's "bedpan" doctrine. As the architect of the NHS put it, "When a bedpan is dropped on a hospital floor, its noise should resound in the Palace of Westminster". I suspect that his successors have all wished that it didn't. But parliamentary accountability means, in effect, that the Secretary of State is at least notionally answerable for everything that happens in the NHS. Westminster is the great amplifier of discontent at the periphery, though in recent years this role has to an extent been taken over by the media; dropped bedpans are now the staple of television coverage.

Centralisation, further, feeds on itself. Successive secretaries of state have sought to distance themselves from what happens on the ground; devolving blame, as it were, to individual health authorities if resources have to be rationed while centralising credit for anything good that happens. But the need to account for public money inevitably drags responsibility back to the centre. Hence the recurring cycle of attempted devolution followed by a return to centralisation that has characterised the NHS over the decades. Whenever ministers have sought to distance themselves from day to day involvement in the running of the NHS – for example, by the creation of the NHS Executive – they have soon been forced back into taking a day to day interest in its affairs, ranging from hospital closures to drawing the boundaries of health authorities.

No wonder, then, that successive secretaries of states of both parties have been attracted by the notion of an independent health care commission; a conclusion usually drawn, however, in their memoirs once they had left office. Similarly, they have pondered, if only in internal memoranda on the possibility of divorcing NHS funding from taxation, of finding some sort of independent source of finance. The two, of course, go together. And while NHS funding continues to come out of general revenue, the idea of spinning off a health care commission is in my view likely to remain a mirage.

Responsibility without control

The responsibility of ministers is, however, of a peculiar kind. It is, to a large extent, responsibility without direct control. Ministers do not employ health authorities' managers, though they appoint the various boards. And they certainly do not employ doctors. There is thus a gap between accountability for the resources provided and control over how those resources are used in practice. The result has been that as the political costs of keeping a tight lid on NHS spending have risen, so attempts to strengthen control have increased. If there is public dissatisfaction with the performance of the NHS and if increasing funding is ruled out as a policy option for dealing with such dissatisfaction, then the answer has always been "increase efficiency". And for the past 15 years at least, increasing efficiency has been equated with stronger management, as well as introduction of a mimic market, a Thatcher "reform" that grew from a little publicised report in 1985 by a visiting American academic, Professor Alain Enthoven.

109

But the drive for ever greater productivity, for squeezing ever more activity out of the budget, in turn produced another twist in the story. It has caused resentment among the medical profession. Not only do doctors see themselves losing power to managers,   but they also feel that their professional autonomy is being eroded. Evidence based medicine, as propounded by the Department of Health, may be highly desirable but it can also become a tool of control if translated into purchasing plans restricting the freedom of doctors to determine their own patterns of practice.

The evidence on all these points is ambiguous. Anyway, I am unclear to what extent the perceived loss of power and erosion of autonomy are real or imagined. In many respects the profession has been remarkably successful in guarding its autonomy. We have to look only at the extent of external control exercised in the United States over the activities of doctors and contrast this with the ability of the British profession to ensure that any

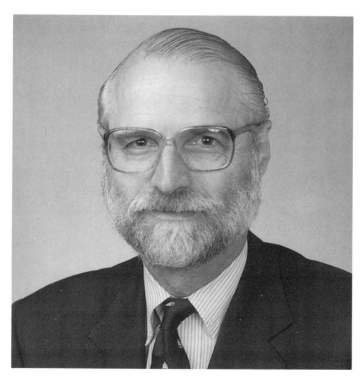

Professor Alain Enthoven. A distinguished American health economist, his monograph *Reflections on the Managment of the NHS*, published in 1985 by the Nuffield Provincial Hospitals Trust, was to influence greatly the Conservative Government's review of the NHS in 1988-9.

scrutiny is carried out by peers. But, for the purposes of this argument, the crucial point is that the medical profession *feels* increasingly resentful. In other words, the political costs of the NHS are likely to increase. Not only is disgruntlement likely to feed the inbuilt tendency to "denigration", it is also undermining the willingness of doctors to disguise resource constraints as clinical decisions.

The future

- Governments will be seeking a system that is more pluralistic and diverse both in its sources of funding and in the distribution of responsibility for the delivery of health care.
- This prospect should not provoke alarm since the ideals that shaped the NHS in 1948 – the collective assumption of responsibility for the equitable delivery of health care – have served us well and remain the benchmarks for testing any proposals for reform.
- The institutional architecture of the NHS was designed in an era of faith in centralisation and professional paternalism; the structure may no longer be appropriate in a changing society.

The balance sheet is therefore changing as political costs threaten to outweigh the economic benefits of the NHS to governments. My hunch is therefore that the political odds against radical reform are also changing. Whatever the ideology of the government in power, the search will be on for a system of funding or governance that insulates politicians more from professional and public pressures, a system more pluralistic and diverse in its sources of funding and in the distribution of responsibility for the delivery of health care. It is not a prospect, in my view, that need cause alarm. The ideals that shaped the NHS in 1948 remain the benchmarks for testing any proposal for reform. But the institutional architecture of the NHS, designed in an era of faith in centralisation and paternalism, may no longer be appropriate.

19: Why and how did the BMA come to love the NHS?

Stephen Lock

I started at the *British Medical Journal* in 1964, to be flabbergasted by the attitude of my medical editorial colleagues towards the NHS. Without exception, they regarded it as a temporary aberration, which any minute would be replaced by an alternative system. Such feelings reminded me of the early novels of Nicolas Nabokov, of down at heel exiled White Russians waiting for the Czar's return so that they could return from the Côte d'Azure to their vast estates in the Ukraine. And, down-at-heelness excepted, perhaps the comparison was not all that fanciful, given that the editor, Hugh Clegg, who had personally written all the editorials arguing against the NHS, was married to a delightful baroness from Smolensk.

So were these five doctors merely out of touch? Two had never practised in the health service, two only very briefly, and the fifth had worked largely in the pharmaceutical industry. Nevertheless, all were very much in touch with an important section of medical thought: the medicopoliticians – those in the royal colleges and especially those in the central BMA. And medicopolitics bulked very much larger at the *BMJ* then than they have since. We know how relieved many doctors were by the introduction of the NHS. A community physician once told me of his general practitioner parents' joy at a year of bad debts wiped out overnight, while a survey on the tenth anniversary showed most doctors in favour. Even so, the backdrop of dissatisfaction must have been sufficient to make many regard the service as ripe for radical change or even replacement by something totally different.

How attitudes had changed by 1991, when I finished at the *BMJ* ! By then, we had doctors fighting in public to preserve the NHS. Nor were such battles confined to the BMA though, through its Chairman of Council, John Marks, and a lively press office, the association had run a highly outspoken campaign, with large posters on public hoardings attacking the

Secretary of State for Health. The academics had talked of an imminent crisis, lobbying for better funded research and teaching, while the presidents of three medical royal colleges had not only issued a statement about underfunding of the NHS (an unusual step for the apolitical colleges) but had also had a sticky interview with the Prime Minister herself.

When and how had such radical change in professional policy come about? To answer this with academic rigour would need a formidable amount of time, with access to a wide variety of records. Thus, since 1980 Charles Webster has been writing the official history of the NHS: his first volume (479 pages) took us to 1957 and the second (988 pages), published last year, to 1979. Without tongue in cheek he states that: ". . . this survey does not pretend to offer a comprehensive review of health care during the period under consideration". And all historians have their own ideas of when the record changes from journalism to history, warning about writing about recent events with any roundness or fairness, let alone objectivity.

Doctors' changing views, as reflected in the *BMJ*

In trying to answer when and why the profession changed its attitude from grudging acceptance to blatant defence and pleas for betterment, I chose journalism and largely one source, the *BMJ*. For the first 40 years of the NHS, my period here, this reported the principal documents and debates on the major issues and crucially the latter at the BMA's annual "parliament": the Annual Representative Meeting (ARM). I therefore skimmed through every volume of the *BMJ* from the introduction of the NHS to 40 years later, using the ARM debates as the major indicator of what many doctors felt.

Initially, debates concentrated on pay and conditions: the right to private practice, the bane of frivolous night calls, and fees for lectures to nurses, for instance. To be sure, in 1954, there were complaints of delays in outpatient departments and one comment that: "It appears that the service at present provided is not equal to the demands made upon it". But it took the celebrations of the tenth anniversary of the NHS for more specific complaints to be made. One representative at the ARM pointed out that non-urgent cases in Manchester had to wait for three to four years before being admitted to hospital, while another commented that not even two completely new hospitals had been built since the NHS had begun.

Nevertheless, primarily these years were spent in negotiating changes in the service conditions and remuneration of doctors, particularly general practitioners (GPs), with the Dankwerts award righting some anomalies in 1952 and the setting up of the Royal Commission on Doctors' and Dentists' Remuneration. But the subsequently established independent review body on pay did not quieten the rumblings of discontent among GPs about the pool method of payments in the late 1950s and early 1960s (p84).

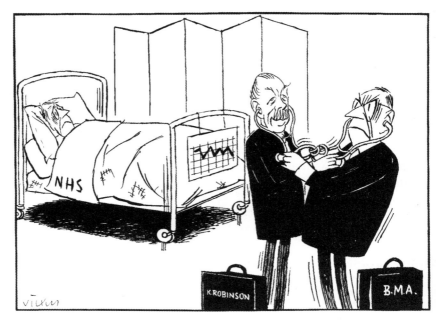

Cartoonist Vicky's view of the standoff in 1965 between the BMA and Kenneth Robinson over the future of general practice. Reproduction with permission from the Solo Syndication and Literary Agency.

These surfaced slowly but were forcibly expressed in a letter to the *BMJ*, in 1963. The authors, partners in a Winchester practice, already had many of the features subsequently regarded as the norm of good practice: attached ancillary staff, undergraduate training, and hospital attachments for the partners – all introduced at their own expense but "with the minimum of encouragement from the Ministry of Health". The pool system, which averaged expenses reimbursed to GPs regardless of the quality of premises, facilities or supporting staff, was a serious disincentive to good practice. This same year a new group, the General Practitioners' Association, was established to ginger up the BMA and two years later a turbulent ARM at Swansea responded with calls for an item of service based contract and the launch of an alternative, Independent Medical Services, to be funded by insurance contributions from patients. Protracted negotiations between Kenneth Robinson, Minister of Health, and Jim Cameron, Chairman of the BMA's GP Committee, on the Family Doctors' Charter finally settled the major disquiet in general practice in 1966 and led to its renaissance.

Focus on hospitals' problems

Thereafter attention largely centred on hospitals, focusing, for example, on long waiting lists, poor standards in psychiatric hospitals, and fears that kidney transplants might be being restricted on financial grounds while in 1970 Henry Miller, a shrewd and witty Professor of Medicine, told an ARM of his utter conviction that a shortage of money lay at the heart of the NHS troubles. And the 1970s were to be characterised not only by high inflation and government measures to reduce it, with an inevitable deleterious effect on the NHS, but also by industrial action by hospital ancillary staff. Initially, the latter were determined on getting Labour policy on abolishing private practice in hospitals implemented and, subsequently, that their pay should breach the official limits. As a result of all these troubles, in 1979 Jim Cameron, by then the Chairman of the BMA Council, could claim that idealism in the NHS had been dissipated. "The most fundamental problems are to be found within our hospitals," he told the ARM. "Surely a waiting list of nearly three-quarters of a million is a sufficient sign of impending disaster."

Thus, the celebrations of the 30th anniversary were low key and in the subsequent decade the ARM's concern grew steadily and its tone became increasingly shrill. In 1980, Tony Grabham, Cameron's successor, commented that the NHS was far from being comprehensive. Britain was so far behind other countries that it had not even legislated on car seat belts. No fewer than 33 motions at that meeting concerned cuts, funding, and resource allocation, a principal composite motion reading, "That this meeting expresses its grave concern at the financial problems facing the NHS and in particular its effect on nursing staffing and the inevitable consequences on patient care". And over the next few years NHS funding occupied the meetings more and more, particularly in the chairman's opening review which, with Grabham and subsequently John Marks, became a key focus for the press reports. A year before the NHS's 40th anniversary, the presidents of the three principal medical royal colleges made one of their rare public statements: alternative and additional funding must be found, they emphasised, calling on the government to save the NHS. All this culminated, outside the period I am considering, in Mrs Thatcher's imposition of yet a further reorganisation of the NHS (in the form of an internal market) and in the BMA's public campaign for increased funding, with a public debate which continues and as I write is getting even more shrill.

Watershed in doctors' attitude to the NHS

So much for the facts; what about their analysis? Clearly there are several interpretations, but few would argue against a kind of watershed around 1979–1981, after which things were different. The narrow interpretation

115

would explain the changes by personalities. Around this time both the chairmanship of council and the secretaryship of the BMA changed. Tony Grabham was a warmhearted general surgeon whose job at a peripheral hospital had forced him to face the impact of shortages. In contrast, his consultant predecessor, Walpole Lewin, was a reserved neurosurgeon from a teaching hospital, where perhaps shortages were less evident. Some might also argue that John Havard, the BMA's shrewd Secretary, did not need to be as obsessed with general practitioners' problems as his predecessors and could concentrate on hospital difficulties.

The structural interpretation would argue that the BMA had reversed its falling membership in the 1950s by tackling the thornier, if easier, difficulties of general practice and so could then turn to the hospitals. Consultants have always been more divided among themselves – a reflection of the specialty loyalties – than family doctors, with their coherent organisational and negotiating structure that predated the NHS. It was some years after the NHS had started before the BMA could become solely responsible for consultants' terms and conditions of service after the royal colleges had learnt that as charities they could not take on trade union responsibilities. As for hospital junior doctors, for many years their views had been largely subordinated to those of consultants. The 1970s, however, saw them break through the BMA's traditional hierarchy and develop medicopolitical parity with their seniors in the association.

Nevertheless, there is a simpler interpretation altogether. For by the watershed, consultants had begun to realise that the hospital service would stay as underfunded as ever. They had accepted that the first 30 years had been spent in extending specialist services and developing new ones; in 1962 the government had promised to spend £500 million on new buildings over ten years and there had been recurrent financial crises. Now, however, things had changed. The promised hospitals had not been built, waiting lists were getting even longer, yet the government still seemed to concentrate on the relatively cheap general practice and other needs cited in a new priorities document: those of the elderly and handicapped, the mentally ill, maternity, and neonatal care.

To go to richer countries was to be reminded of what could be achieved – handsome new buildings and proportionately more lifesaving procedures, such as dialysis and coronary artery bypass surgery. Yet hospital consultants were hardly popular in the community, partly as a legacy of their industrial action during confrontation with the government over more work sensitive contracts and private practice in the 1970s; partly because Ian Kennedy's influential Reith lectures questioned their hegemony, while the Black Report of 1979 had instanced the effects of poverty on health (p21); and partly because of a new radical critique by Arthur Seldon of the Institute of Economic Affairs arguing that the NHS had failed not because of remediable defects in its organisation or finance but because of fundamental flaws in its conception. Add to that an obdurate Prime Minister who was tackling trade unions and special interest groups head on, was introducing business style management into the NHS, and was armed with Treasury evidence of continual waste in the NHS (particularly in hospital planning) and the scene was set, I believe, for yet further escalation of dissatisfaction, which persists today. Such professional dissatisfaction erodes morale and commitment which, coupled with other factors (see box), makes me gloomy about the NHS's future.

The future

Though primary care is a success, the hospital service in particular will continue to deteriorate, given the following factors.

- Politicians' reluctance to spend more of the gross domestic product on the NHS (the money could readily be hypothecated for cost effectiveness, such as more intensive care beds and life enhancing operations, such as hip and cataract surgery.
- The new government maintaining the tradition of appointing to the health department a lacklustre politician at the end of a career and immediately finding money for such ridiculous imperial extravagances as atomic submarines and fighter aircraft.
- An absence of any new thinking in the recent general elections.
- Crucially, the fall in the national bed numbers to under 300,000.

Finally, the failure of debates on rationing elsewhere in the developed world suggests that these would be no more successful in Britain. Nevertheless, the failure of the NHS in the 1990s lies in every one of us, in our obsession with two irreconcilable opposites: Nordic levels of social services and American levels of taxation.

20: Medicine and medicopolitics: a personal saga

John Marks

The National Health Service started on the day I qualified in Edinburgh. Ten days later I went back to St Leonard's Hospital, Hoxton, where I had spent time as a student, to tell them the news. I was offered a locum post, starting immediately (the preregistration year had not yet been invented). That night, a 90 year old man was admitted with acute retention. I was the anaesthetist! Both of us survived. Medicine has come a long way since then.

After house jobs and National Service, I came home to massive medical unemployment, so I drove a lorry until I got a job as houseman in obstetrics and gynaecology in Bath. There my career plan to be a consultant obstetrician ended. I was told, rightly, that I had ten thumbs, and should rethink my future, so I became a trainee in general practice. In those days, when a hospital career was generally seen as the road to professional success, many entrants to general practice were trainee specialists who had lost out in the fierce competition for senior hospital posts. Anyway, there I was on a salary of £750, with plenty of day and night work and minimal training. On the positive side I became a "Founder Associate" of the nascent College of General Practitioners.

With two years as a full-time assistant behind me I applied, with 119 others, for a partnership in Borehamwood. By the standards of the day it was a superb practice with decent premises, receptionists, a secretary, and its own clinics. I was offered the job, to start six weeks before my planned wedding. There were conditions: firstly, we had to abandon our honeymoon; secondly, I would wait seven years for parity; and thirdly, the practice would lease two premises, each owned by a partner's wife, for 30 years at double the realistic rent. I accepted. The alternative was to emigrate, as did a third of my student cohort. My anger over the exploitation of doctors by the State, and particularly by other doctors, that I saw and experienced then remains with me to this day.

The practice served a developing London County Council estate.

Almost every patient had medical and social problems and we could register up to 20 such families a day. Hospital services at Barnet and Edgware could not cope and we did about a 100 home confinements a year. A night in bed was a rarity and our enormous workload was a source of wonderment, and sometimes disbelief, to other doctors.

The senior partner made medical educational films, so it became policy that the group should allow its members to do things not related to conventional general practice. That attitude allowed me to do sessions as a clinical assistant, to become a divisional surgeon in the St John's Ambulance service, and to enter medicopolitics. The real drop in our already relatively low income was a price worth paying for these extraneous activities.

In 1959 my wife joined the practice on even worse terms but by 1964, when our senior partner gave up medicine, Britain was experiencing a shortage of doctors. We "persuaded" a doctor to return from abroad and the laws of supply and demand gave him a very good deal. The practice continued to grow in numbers of patients and doctors until, by the time I retired, there were nine partners, five men and four women, caring for 16,500 patients.

Before the medicopolitical crisis of 1964, GPs were paid solely by capitation, through a fixed "pool" of government controlled funds, which included averaged expenses. That resulted in progressive practices subsidising a large number of low quality ones, often run by older doctors hankering after the "good old days" – namely, before the NHS. Too many did well financially while providing barely acceptable standards of care.

Crisis in general practice: I enter medicopolitics

The intense anger among GPs which followed the fifth report of the review body in 1964 galvanised the BMA's General Medical Services Committee (GMSC), which represented all NHS GPs, into producing a Charter for General Practice or Family Doctors' Charter, as it was commonly called. It also led to my first involvement in medicopolitics at a national level. I had been elected to the Hertfordshire Local Medical Committee by my colleagues in Borehamwood and Elstree, and in 1965 I became vice-chairman. A special conference of LMCs met to discuss the proposed radical new contract for GPs. The suggested direct reimbursement of rents and 70% of staff wages was of great import to the relatively young doctors of Hertfordshire. We agreed to support a motion calling for that part of the "new deal" to be implemented forthwith. Our usual representative declined to speak to it and I went to BMA House in his place. Needless to say, the platform persuaded the meeting to "pass to the next business", an early lesson for me in conference procedures.

In those days the Conference of LMCs and the BMA's Representative Body debated the same issues separately, sometimes producing conflicting decisions. My path to the Representative Body from the Barnet Division was blocked by the local member of the BMA Council, who labelled me a "communist" because I had the effrontery to support the NHS. He left the area, but still thought he represented the Barnet Division. The members took a different view. They sent me to the association's Special Representative Meeting which followed the conference, where my credentials were challenged by my predecessor, supported by the then secretary of the BMA, Dr Derek Stevenson, an influential figure. I convinced Derek that he was wrong and that summer I attended my first Annual Representative Meeting in Exeter. I soon realised that to move general practice, and the BMA, in what I thought was the right direction, I needed to be on the BMA Council and the GMSC but my paths to both were blocked.

Beating the system to lead a double life

The GMSC was elected in part on a regional basis by groups. Hertfordshire, Bedfordshire, Southend on Sea, North East London, and Essex LMCs made up "group S". The last two had been one until 1964 and had a cosy arrangement to support each other's candidates. Three successive defeats made me determined to beat the system so in 1968 I wrote a second, private, election address to LMC members outside the Essex cabal, pointing out that if they used their two votes I could never oust the incumbents. They used one and I became a new member of the GMSC with John Ball, Brian Whowell, Benny Alexander, and Gyles Riddle, all of whom became leaders of the profession.

At that time the BMA Council was elected in part by members in regions and in part by the Representative Body. At the latter, a "northern block" controlled the elections. I was a southerner and two respected "elder statesmen" held the local seats and seemed unassailable. However, one retired in 1973 and I won the local election. Had anyone suggested that one day I would chair the Council I would have recommended psychiatric treatment. Cockney, Jewish, grammar school general practitioners were not "the right material".

After that election I had a double life, but the clinical and medicopolitical parts had many links. Rightly so, for I had been elected to represent practising doctors. In 1966, after the passing of David Steel's Abortion Act but before its implementation, I sent Betty, a nice young mother, to a local gynaecologist. While waiting for her appointment she became pregnant. The consultant gave her a letter, which Betty opened, telling me that she would not terminate the pregnancy, though the question had not been raised. Betty bought a Higginson's syringe, douched herself, and died on the bathroom floor. Thirty years later I can still see her there.

Incredibly, BMA policy was that though so called "social" abortion was legal, it was unethical. To change that policy led to people like me being condemned as Trotskyists and murderers by the "pro-lifers". Ultimately the reformers won, the representatives deciding that the Act was a "practical and humane piece of legislation". Later, on the association's behalf, I helped to defeat the Corrie, Brain, and other parliamentary bills which tried to turn the clock back.

Top of the agenda at the BMA's Annual Meeting of 1969 was the question of heart transplants. Before I left home one of my children (Richard, now a consultant anaesthetist) had said to me: "Daddy, of course heart transplants must go on. When I'm your age, one case will be a brain transplant and the other a heart transplant". I quoted Richard's words to the meeting, adding that "It may be years before we have a successful heart transplant. We may never have one, but we can't deny the public the possibility of it." Supporters of transplantation won the debate, the press quoted my speech extensively, and I learnt the value of soundbites.

Reform of the General Medical Council

In 1970, a Special Representative Meeting was called to endorse the BMA Council's decision to accept a demand from the General Medical Council (GMC) for an annual retention fee. A motion proposed by me, that such payment should be conditional on the majority of the members of the GMC being directly elected by the medical profession, was carried by a huge majority. As a result, I found myself Joint Chairman of the BMA Committee which gave evidence to the government initiated inquiry into regulation of the profession, chaired by Alec Merrison, a university vice chancellor. Later I was deeply involved in consultations on the Bill which became the Medical Act of 1978. Subsequently I was elected to the reformed GMC.

The GMC's constitution having been radically restructured, the Representative Body turned to the BMA's constitution, inviting an industrialist, Sir Paul Chambers, to do an independent inquiry into the association's structure. Reporting in March 1972, he recommended a streamlining of the association's structure and the abolition of the GMSC and other autonomous "craft committees". In November the Representative Body accepted "Chambers in principle" and the association almost tore itself apart, with the craft committees fiercely resisting any loss of their autonomy within the BMA. After much manoeuvring I successfully proposed a motion at the annual meeting in Folkestone reversing that decision after a roll call vote, the first time this had happened in living memory.

Kenneth Clarke's bombshell

Gradually ascending the medicopolitical ladder, I was elected chairman of the Representative Body in 1981 and Chairman of Council in July 1984. That November Kenneth Clarke, then Minister for Health, gave the association two hours' notice of the Secretary of State's intention to introduce a limited list of NHS drugs. This was despite undertakings given to Parliament the previous year not to do so and despite a long tradition of ministers consulting with the profession in advance of proposals for changes in the NHS. The BMA, believing that such restrictions were not in patients' interests, opposed this bombshell change. It failed miserably, but we learnt lessons, particularly about publicity, which we used later.

In December 1988, Mrs Thatcher suddenly announced on television, not to the House of Commons, a "review" of the NHS. On 31 January 1989 Kenneth Clarke, by then Secretary of State, launched the misnamed White

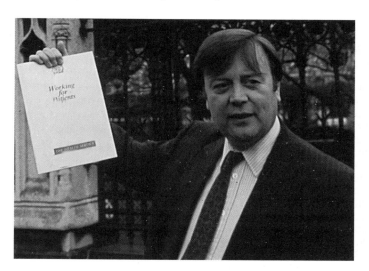

Kenneth Clarke. He replaced John Moore as Secretary of State in August 1989 at a critical point in Prime Minister Thatcher's review of the NHS. Here, Mr Clarke holds up the outcome of that top level review: the White Paper *Working for Patients,* published on 31 January 1989. The controversial proposals include splitting purchasers from providers of services, giving general practitioners the funds to purchase cetain secondary care services and making the NHS more consumer sensitive. Reproduced with permission from Rex Features.

Paper *Working for Patients* in a blaze of media glory, which contrasted dramatically with the secrecy surrounding its preparation. It proposed an unknown, untested "internal market" for the NHS, based on self-governing hospitals and budget holding GPs. I announced that the BMA would consult its members before making any statement. Kenneth Clarke's speeches, however, had already been written and the next morning, without any evidence, he unjustifiably accused the BMA of opposing all change in the NHS.

The BMA's Council issued a report and meetings of members all over the country discussed it. The response was massive. Doctors, realising that the NHS and patient care were in danger, instructed their leaders to oppose the changes and, more importantly, to inform the public of their views. The council set up a special working party, labelled by the media "The BMA War Party", which met at least fortnightly. We did not conform to the fuddy-duddy image of the BMA which Clarke and others cherished. Several of us had acquired the skills to promote our cause in the media and elsewhere. We met many MPs, mainly Tory, and debated the issues at the Oxford Union and elsewhere, while thousands of GPs distributed leaflets in their waiting rooms.

The BMA today

The Trade Union Act of 1971 forced the BMA to become a trade union. It led to members of Council being directly elected by the members in constituencies. Scotland, Wales and Northern Ireland each have a "national" seat and there are four open to all doctors in the United Kingdom. Constituencies exist for doctors in various "crafts" and these are further subdivided between "United Kingdom" and "regional" seats. Competition for the national seats at the UK level is intense and to a lesser degree for the craft national seats, but the vast majority of regional members, mainly senior participants in BMA committees, are elected unopposed. However, over the years the increased number of younger members – medical students and doctors in training – serving on BMA committees has immeasurably improved the quality of debates.

Unfortunately the number of members who bother to vote in Council elections is abysmally low, with an average turnout below 30%. I believe this reflects apathy and demoralisation, not unreserved support for the establishment. Elections for the GMC and for the President of the Royal College of General Practitioners produce similarly low polls. The standing of the Representative Body and the standard of its debates have also improved. In part, this is a result of informed chairmanship, the hiving off of much "trade union" material to the craft conferences, and also the power of the Annual Meeting's Agenda Committee to produce composite motions, allocate debating times and, above all, to prioritise issues. Now, the Representative Body is seen and accepted as the "Parliament of the Profession", and not an elderly gentlemen's talking shop, as it was in my early days in medicopolitics.

The association spent a large sum on advertising, most of it excellent. We won the battle of minds, as shown by a series of opinion polls and other evidence. We lost the war to an arrogant government with a large majority. Sadly, all of our predictions came true.

I have now retired from practice and largely from medicopolitics and find it difficult to forecast the NHS's future. Perhaps the damage inflicted by the last government is irreparable. The Labour Government intends to resuscitate the service, but seems reluctant to tell the public the truth: if Britain wants a high quality NHS, the country must spend much more of the national financial cake on it.

21:   I've never known times as bad: an Ulster perspective

Graeme McDonald

In the early hours of the morning, I was in the anaesthetic room being prepared for an emergency laparotomy and what would turn out to be a sigmoid colectomy for cancer. Nights spent reading the findings of the *Confidential Enquiry into Peri-operative Deaths* led to some anxiety until I discovered that a consultant surgeon and a consultant anaesthetist were present. The anaesthetist introduced himself by saying, "I remember you – we were on the same Lego building team at that management course".

I have been a participant in the National Health Service as a patient, a psychiatrist, and a junior medicopolitician. Competing to build the highest tower of Lego was not the most pointless thing in which I became involved. Reflecting on my experiences of the service from different perspectives produced several common themes.

When I started at medical school I had, like most others, no realistic knowledge of what lay before me. The NHS was barely a quarter of a century old. The Labour government was fighting with consultants about pay beds and losing. Junior doctors were taking industrial action to win marginal improvements in their lot. The sausage machine of undergraduate medical education led me to believe that every problem had a solution and that the service could provide all necessary treatment free of charge to patients according to clinical need.

I entered my houseman's year with apprehension but became the tired, sometimes uncaring, automaton who professed absolute confidence in his own knowledge and skills. The dehumanising structure caused me to lose sight of the purpose of medicine. Participation in medicopolitics gave me a simple creed:

- more spending leads to a better service;
- medical manpower should be planned so that wasteful blockages are removed;

125

- hospitals should be bigger and more centralised;
- consultants should work harder.

In the years that have passed since, just about every assumption has proved to be ill founded. As a patient of several hospital departments, I learnt that senior house officers would diagnose my various problems quickly and with certainty. The only disadvantage of this was that they were often wrong. The more senior the practitioner I consulted, the more likely I was to be given expressions of uncertainty. A consultant dermatologist examining a skin rash told me, "I'm not sure what it is – if it's still there in six weeks it will probably be due to the cancer".

In 1988 I returned from a visit to the then Soviet Socialist Republic of the Ukraine, where perhaps the most striking impression was to see a fully equipped modern hospital – built with aid to help with the consequences of the Chernobyl nuclear accident – apparently being used for the treatment of wealthy foreigners flown in to stay in the adjoining hotel. The following day I led the negotiating team of the BMA's Junior Doctors Committee in presenting evidence to the profession's pay review body. The script was familiar. I explained that junior doctors, exploited by consultants and managers, had never worked harder and that their morale had never been lower. I added the obvious conclusion that only a substantial increase in juniors' income could hope to remedy these problems. A professor of industrial relations from Wales replied, "Young man, for as long as I've been sitting on this side of the table I've heard doctors' leaders complaining that times have never been as bad. I appreciate that you have to say so but let's get on to the evidence".

Psychiatric services under stress

At the outset of the NHS in 1948, psychiatry as a science was in its infancy. Large asylums were expanding in capacity, drug treatments were few and ineffective, and a limited range of psychotherapies was available only in private practice. Apparently bizarre treatments such as insulin coma therapy and mutilating psychosurgery continued into the 1960s. It is arguable whether community care was made possible by the advent of effective antipsychotic drugs or a change in professional attitudes. Whatever the origin, the policy cannot be said to have been a complete success. Too often efforts to secure care in the community have shown that the community does not care.

Northern Ireland has been fortunate in having strong family networks, little population mobility and, unlike the rest of the UK, integration of health and social services both before the 1991 structural changes and since then within both purchasers and providers. We have been fortunate to avoid the appalling problems of London's mental health services. In the capital, long stay beds have closed without adequate aftercare being arranged. A

126

vast population of mobile, homeless, psychotic, drug abusing patients move from service to service with little prospect of continuity of care. The use of NHS inpatient facilities is restricted to psychotic patients. Many patients are detained under mental health legislation in unpleasant and antitherapeutic settings. A shortage of beds means that patients can find themselves briefly admitted to a sequence of hospitals in both the public and private sectors. The criminal justice system expensively accommodates and further disables many of those who need care.

A succession of suicides and homicides lead to expensive inquiries that conclude that better communication between staff would reduce the risks. The structures and facilities that would enable such communication remain as distant as ever. It becomes difficult to recruit candidates for previously prestigious academic psychiatry posts. Staff of all disciplines feel that they are made scapegoats for the failures in mental health care. That and the lack of support have led to a rapid turnover of staff. The surprise is that so much is achieved in these circumstances.

In recent years, Northern Ireland has become accustomed to delegations of managers from England visiting to see the benefits of health and social services integration. There seems little doubt that keeping the petty jealousies and rivalries in the same office can minimise harm to patients. However, those who see simply a change in administrative structures as the answer to the problems of psychiatric care in London are misguided. Integration of health and social care is wise but does little to solve the structural and funding problems. The techniques of evidence based medicine have much to teach politicians and managers. Until this happens we can expect many more mission statements, corporate logos, and untoward incident inquiries.

Northern Ireland's troubles

Working as a psychiatrist in Northern Ireland has its own difficulties. I work in a sector of about 60,000 people. Unemployment is endemic. The area contains people of one tribal group only. Young men have found the temptations of political violence irresistible. Imprisonment, mutilation or premature death are more likely outcomes than glorious success. The ill educated youth of Great Britain's inner cities joins the army to see the world and finds itself looking down a gun barrel at its counterparts in Belfast. A reciprocal brutality gives each group justification for continued atrocity.

The press responds to violence with the assertion that perpetrators are psychotic or psychopathic. My contact with the men and women involved has revealed singlemindedness, determination, and self-belief rather than delusional thought. In contrast to so-called ordinary, decent criminals, the politically violent tend to have a good educational background, to have been brought up in a stable home, and rarely to abuse intoxicants. However misguided their actions seem, they are not caused by mental illness. The exception to this somewhat rosetinted view is seen as the politicians call ceasefires. Once societies are immersed in the culture of violence it is difficult to withdraw. Organisations previously dedicated to fighting a clear and common enemy become brutal enforcers of community justice. Profiting from drug dealing alternates with the mutilation through shooting and beatings of those at the bottom of the social hierarchy who are not part of the organisation.

The present political violence began in 1969. Paradoxically, the mental health of populations exposed to violence initially improved. Suicide rates declined as homicide rates rose. Prescription of psychotropic drugs fell. The fight against a clearly recognised common enemy did much for community cohesion. This cohesion was further developed by migration to single religion areas separated by "peace lines". With the passage of time the common problems of poverty, unemployment, and relationship difficulties broke through the community spirit and continued to cause many more psychological problems than political violence ever did. The violence, with little evidence of success, persisted alongside rising suicide rates and ever greater uptake of mental health services. A striking finding has been the psychological resilience of people exposed to the most horrific experiences. The frequency with which mainland colleagues diagnose post-traumatic stress disorder in patients with normal emotional reactions to mild or moderate emotional trauma is perplexing.

Practitioners in the province have had to learn to cope with the ethics of dealing with patients who acknowledge that they have committed murder but have been undetected or who have been tortured by government or illegal agencies.

Unchanging nature of medicopolitics

As in politics in Northern Ireland, medicopolitics has changed little. An attempt to date the proceedings of the BMA's Junior Doctors Committee by the subjects under discussion would prove futile. The aims have been straightforward: to expand consultant numbers so that doctors spend four times as long in the consultant grade as in training; to reduce junior doctors' hours of work to a safe minimum; to ensure doctors reach the apex of their abilities; and to improve postgraduate medical education. The evidence of history and common sense suggests that no two of these can be achieved together. The inertia of the system has meant that each bit of central tinkering has led to an equal and opposite response and thus to restoration of the equilibrium. *Achieving a Balance** led to a rate of consultant expansion little different to that which preceded it and a renaming of junior jobs to escape the definitions in the agreement. The *New Deal* on hours of work, intended to reduce juniors' heavy workloads (an enduring NHS problem), led to many doctors believing that they were working more hours with less continuity of care and for less money.

Junior doctor politicians represent but are not always representative of their colleagues. Those who occupy leadership positions often find themselves more distant from their colleagues than from those they oppose in negotiations. Having negotiated a deal, the leadership finds it hard to secure support from their constituents. Implementation is followed by a prolonged period of backtracking. Cardiac surgeons are allowed to choose to work longer hours for training purposes, research jobs are excluded from manpower calculations or limits on staff grade numbers are found to be unduly restrictive. It is but a matter of time until the presently expanding consultant grade becomes divided into two tiers. As the equilibrium is restored, the cycle of discontent begins again.

The future

- The NHS will enter the next half century as it entered the last: inadequately funded, providing inequitable services, and striving to cope with insoluble problems.
- It will be impossible to provide for everyone a comprehensive health and illness service, free of charge and available when needed.
- Ways to decide priorities, ration care, and charge patients will have to be found.

The "establishment" seems to require a group of people who will do the work but not expect to reach the privileged ranks of those who run the system. At different times this group seems to have been identified as immigrants from the Indian subcontinent, women, and perpetual senior house officers. The system constantly tries to create a permanent subconsultant grade. Experience shows that the appointment of an additional consultant to a service rarely reduces the workload of those already in post. Instead, a new empire is steadily built, consuming resources and expanding in a futile bid to meet the infinite demand. As the empire grows, complaints of overwork and unmet needs lead to the budding of a new consultant post.

The 50th anniversary of the founding of the NHS offers an opportunity to reflect. The certainties and good intentions of its founders have proved,

---

* (a joint government/profession report in 1986 on the balance between the numbers of doctors in training and numbers of consultants.)

with the wisdom of hindsight, to be optimistic. The service will enter the next half century as it entered the last: inadequately funded, providing inequitable services, and striving to cope with insoluble problems. At a time when spending levels are high and treatment options broader than ever, many doctors claim that times have never been as bad. I do not see how the government can provide a comprehensive health and illness service, free of charge and available at the time of need to the whole population of the United Kingdom. Difficult decisions about priorities, treatments, and charging patients lie ahead. At the core of the service is the individual confidential transaction between the practitioner and the patient. Viewing the service from both sides tells me that if we continue to get that right most of the time, we will have achieved much.

22:   A lost dream

Melanie Phillips

As a journalist, I seem to have been writing the same story about the National Health Service for almost a quarter of a century. In 1974, I wrote in Hemel Hempstead's *Evening Echo* about hospital waiting lists which were out of control and about threadbare services for mentally ill people. In 1994, I wrote in *The Observer* about a total halt to all elective surgery at one London hospital and a chronic shortage of community care.

As time has gone on, however, I have become more rather than less perplexed. We are now receiving medical treatments whose efficacy in improving the quality of our lives could not have been imagined even when I started writing, let alone when the NHS was founded. And yet so many people are in real distress through the failings of the service. My earlier certainty that the root of the problem in the NHS was lack of money has given way to a growing belief that though more money is undoubtedly essential, simply providing more is not the answer either. The problems are broader and more complex.

Looking back through my cuttings books, I find ghostly ancestors of the present rising from their pages. Have we really learnt nothing? In 1974, I reported on a cancer specialist whose clinic was run, as he himself said in passionate despair, like a mass production line, treating highly vulnerable patients like cars or widgets. He was no longer prepared, he said, to work in a state monopoly where it had become impossible to practise medicine properly. The system was now geared to administrators. Patients came last. There were constant complaints that more officials were being appointed than doctors and nurses; there were charges of bureaucratic ossification, passing of bucks and double decision taking. Twenty three years later, a Labour government would come to power pledged *again* to reduce NHS red tape. With every such pledge over the years, the red tape had grown.

In 1975, I reported that impossible demands were being made on the health service in Hertfordshire. Staff at psychiatric hospitals warned that moving patients out into the community would not solve their problems but leave some of them dangerously isolated and less well cared for. In the 1990s, the truth of such warnings became all too visible in the pathetic sights on our streets and in shop doorways. In 1975, an orthopaedic surgeon who had been on call 168 hours per week for 24 years finally revolted when the health authority refused to provide a second surgeon because it had no money to open more operating theatres. "Most of us close our eyes to the conditions we work under," he said.

Those conditions included hospitals where rain poured in through cracks in the roof, operating theatres were closed through burst pipes and infestations of Pharaoh ants, kitchens were condemned by health inspectors, hundreds of patients were crammed into waiting areas where they fell over each other, grimy treatment rooms had flaking paint and brickwork crumbling into equipment. Clearly, there was insufficient money. But looking back, I can see even more clearly that the system was simply unable to respond to what was going on. A consultant radiotherapist wrote to the *Evening Echo*: "The miles and miles of paper grow, our problems multiply and nothing much is done... It is fantastic that these things should be allowed to happen in 1976." How much more fantastic might that doctor have found our even more baroque situation 20 years later?

Secrecy of health authority decisions

Meanwhile, there were constant complaints about the secrecy of health authority decisions and the powerlessness of ordinary people to make their voice heard through the community health councils. I reported on one meeting of the North West Thames Regional Health Authority, which opened at 2.15 pm and was closed to the public at 2.45 pm, with no mention of the cash crisis. Two weeks later, a meeting of the Hertfordshire Area Health Authority opened at 10 am and closed to the public 55 minutes later, only 11 minutes of which had been spent discussing patients; the rest had been on directives, circulars, and how to resist the government's call for administrative economies.

In 1978, I reported for *The Guardian* on the epic fight between the Lambeth, Southwark and Lewisham Health Authority and the Callaghan government. The authority was refusing to impose draconian cuts in its services to balance its budget. Prime Minister Callaghan was said to believe that the crisis in the health service had been exaggerated. But the cash problem had been exacerbated by his own government's policy of redistributing money from "rich" health regions to "poor" ones under the RAWP* formula. Given the parlous state of NHS finances, this actually amounted to redistributing money from the poor to the poor. London was deemed to be "rich" because of all the teaching hospitals; but Lambeth, Southwark and Lewisham were and are some of the most needy boroughs in the country.

The deeply flawed RAWP policy was nevertheless an article of faith

---

* Resource Allocation Working Party, a government appointment body which reported in September 1976. (p62)

among health bureaucrats and planners. It was given particular potency because "rich" London was populated by doctors with lucrative Harley Street private practices, whose perceived arrogance helped fuel the profound animosity which led directly to their nemesis under Mrs Thatcher's internal market ten years later. There was a resentful feeling that hospital consultants appeared to be mainly interested in building professional empires in heroic areas of medicine, which would bestow upon them almost godlike status among the public.

The losers were the Cinderella specialties such as geriatrics or mental health. So it followed that administrators, who had impotently fumed for years about this, came to believe that the public interest resided with themselves in arbitrating between competing interests and securing a fairer distribution of resources. That, however, was the fallacy. Under the internal market, NHS administrators cut a Faustian deal: power to themselves in return for cuts in services, including those so dear to their hearts.

Planning blight

Planning was surely not the solution but an important part of the problem. Equity, that ever moving, indefinable goal of the planners, was always going to be as achievable as the pot of gold buried at the end of the rainbow. Applying formulae derived from moving numbers around bits of paper to messy, real life situations with unpredictable human beings who do not fit neatly into one category was always asking for trouble. Planning meant that small was *not* considered beautiful; giant hospitals replaced "uneconomic" community hospitals. Popular resistance was dismissed as mere sentiment, but the policy was a false economy. Small hospitals had mopped up much social distress, the kind that doesn't register in statistics, which eventually translated itself into intolerable pressures on the giant hospitals' casualty units.

Planners' blight meant "rich" London was deemed to have too many hospital beds. Statistical manipulation wrenched reality to fit the planners' utopian vision of a future in which most surgery would be done in about five seconds flat and with no postoperative problems, the mentally ill could be dispatched into the community and most health care dumped on GPs. In fact, even keyhole surgery requires postoperative care, many mentally ill people cannot cope in the community, and the emphasis on GPs merely stimulated a huge increase in demand for hospital care.

The fact that when the decision was taken to close 15 London hospitals 150,000 people were waiting for hospital treatment in the capital was dismissed as a whingeing irrelevance. The fact that London had already lost thousands of hospital beds during the 1980s was similarly dismissed as yet more special pleading. Once again, the passion for unattainable equality – and for revenge against Sir Lancelot Spratt – was used as an alibi to allow

133

such people to ignore the harsh realities. The result was a nightmare in which GPs were forced to ring round frantically to find a hospital bed anywhere for their desperately ill patients, in which sick people were sent home before they were fully recovered, and in which mentally ill people were abandoned to wander our streets.

No truth for the people

The one thing successive governments could not do was to tell people the truth. Instead, they constructed an ever more fantastic edifice of lies to pretend everything was getting better and better. Health service finances, always byzantine, became so complicated it was virtually impossible to tell whether more money was being spent year by year. How could we tell, when increases turned out to include "efficiency savings", or cuts by another name? The joint imperative to cut costs and pretend more was being achieved was enforced – ironically, given the "independent" trusts – through a highly centralised structure of control. NHS staff were subjected to gagging clauses by a service stuffed with political placemen, whose overriding duty was to keep the lid on the situation and protect it from proper scrutiny. It was an unholy alliance between the free marketeers of the political right and health service professionals who thought they alone were the public interest made flesh.

Putting cost cutting above patients' interests was hardly new. What *was* new were the lengths to which this was taken and the fact that the internal market was a brilliant device which enabled politicians to slough off onto health service managers the responsibility for failing to meet public demand. The result was surgeons standing idle for months because money, supposed to follow the patient, ran out in the first few months of the financial year; patients being decanted from their hospital beds in the middle of the night to make room for new arrivals; and the blood service, that epitome of altruism at the heart of the service, being cut to meet management "efficiency" targets, causing chaos in blood supplies, a reduced service, and danger to patients.

No one in charge

As Conservative health ministers extolled the expanding achievements of the NHS, a friend of mine with a broken leg reported a state of total chaos in her London teaching hospital, with no one appearing to be in charge. There were hardly any nurses and those there were spent much of their time on paperwork. The ward lavatory floors were flooded with urine; pots of excrement were left lying on the bathroom window sill. One overworked orderly was responsible for cleaning, wheeling in meals, and washing up. Throughout her stay, my friend never saw the ward sister. What she did see was an elderly male patient with no pyjama bottoms on, wandering into her cubicle when she was on a bedpan. What she did see, and hear, was a woman dying in loud and intense distress after staff announced that her distraught wails were due to her eating too much, and the woman's relatives walking in unwarned to find her dead in her bed.

Of course, many people have had good experiences of the NHS, which has served them well. Vulnerable members of my own family, however, now live in dread of becoming an inpatient at the local teaching hospital because of their own appalling experiences there. Such things happening to people dear to us, and which we find we have no power to control, tend to alter our perspective on events. Under the internal market, such bad experiences seemed to achieve critical mass. With the increasingly meaningless mantra that health care still remained available free at the point of use, the market was introduced to bring about what ministers did not have the guts to announce upfront, that those who had enough money would make as fast as they could for the independent sector. Two-tierism in health care, glaringly encouraged by GP fundholding, would be extended throughout by default. This is a long, long way from the idealistic intent of a comprehensive, freely available service that inspired Britain in 1948. That dream has been lost.

Challenge for government

- The challenge for the government is to confront the fact that, one way or another, more money needs to be spent on health care.
- This must be raised by either increasing taxes, or developing the commercial and not for profit sectors in a three-way funding partnership with the state.
- If funding were all done through taxes, the problem would surely remain of an authoritarian bureaucracy and the deadly grip of central planners.
- Arguably, an organisation the size of the modern health service is simply unmanageable.
- We should explore ways of developing NHS trusts into institutions on the model of the voluntary hospitals, drawing on our co-operative civic traditions of mutual aid, friendly societies, philanthropy, and trade unions, as well as taxation, to humanise and democratise our hospitals and widen their funding base.
- We must find a way of bringing the NHS down to human size and reconnecting it with local communities who can again feel they own it.
- Only then can we restore the lost principles of the NHS.

23: A district surgeon's seaside perspective

Peter Plumley

The National Health Service was already four years old when I qualified and the hurly burly of the first house job kept my interest focused on patients. The teaching hospital was clean, the nurses were gorgeous, and the porters, impressive in long blue coats with brass buttons, knew all the gossip and goings on. But no one now remembers that the hospital was run by the Brigadier and the Matron. The ward and departmental sisters were, in fact, very senior managers and doctors were guests on the ward, with necessary courtesy on both sides. The junior medical staff, though paid very little, were decently housed and fed. They indulged from time to time in outrageous episodes – but never any that affected patient care.

When I returned as a registrar things were changing, with more of everything, though, with the help of the BMA, the junior staff had negotiated away most of their privileges. The pharmaceutical industry had started the flow of powerful drugs and radiology departments were much larger. The replacement of the Matron by a professor of nursing who believed in management, however, was the harbinger of change. Extra layers of administration and ward sisters in tears made me pleased that my next upward career move was to the south coast.

The Royal East Sussex Hospital, Hastings, was an architect's dream, the worst designed hospital in the UK but beautifully built. It could only have been properly run with a staff two or three times the given establishment. The wards were always full, usually with extra beds, and at the time of my appointment a new hospital was promised. It was cancelled six months later. The second hospital was the old workhouse, mainly filled with medical patients but with a very satisfactory operating theatre.

The third surgical hospital was too large to be called "cottage", but not large enough for a general hospital. When I first saw it, I thought it might be possible to repair a few hernias there. In fact, the people of Bexhill are very proud of their hospital and its League of Friends is probably the most successful in the country. The staff are firmly based in the town and are delightful to work with. For long periods it was a haven of serenity in a sea of dancing bureaucrats.

Summer surge of seaside patients

One of the peculiarities of medicine in a seaside town is that things get busy in the summer. It can almost be guaranteed that one of the patients wishing to be transferred nearer home will come from Aberdeen. Certainly, relations with the ambulance service were strained. But eventually it became obvious, even to South East Thames Regional Health Authority, that the overcrowding was dangerous and we were awarded a race track ward. Prefabricated and flat roofed, these structures lived up to their name. People rushed around and around and the 40 watt bulbs meant we had difficulty recognising the patients postoperatively, but design changes were absolutely forbidden. Then my second hospital planning round passed with eventual cancellation and the money went to Eastbourne!

The South coast of England is known as the Costa Geriatrica, an unkind but apt title. It changed my views of patients entirely. Whereas in London I would write, "this old man of 60", on the coast things are different. Some of the 70 and 80 year olds were moving faster than I did. Age is very much a state of mind and retirement a condition to enjoy. Replacement hips are vastly successful and knee surgery is improving by the year. A good game of golf can be played with two replacement hips and one replacement knee. But moving neighbourhoods to retire is a serious step indeed. Retirement is stressful. Moving house is stressful. Together they can produce a medical disaster in one or even both partners. The presence of a supporting family makes an enormous difference but it remains a critical time in life and retired people need help and understanding. All this influenced how we practised.

The Hospital Management Committee (HMC) was the original governing body of a hospital group. I took my fair share of administration and the HMC was the most fun. It was a collection of local people, most of whom had done a lot of voluntary service and were wise to the operations of central government. This sophisticated approach to public life proved correct in 1974. The new blue, all sparkling, reorganised NHS was supposed to develop its structures by consultation. The south east regional treasurers (aka finance officers or finance controllers)planned a career structure costing half the region's budget. Other departments dreamed similar dreams of power and riches so, as you would expect, the reorganisation was imposed.

Continuous reorganisation

Thereafter, the reorganisation of the NHS became continuous. The HMC was replaced by a small "multidisciplinary" committee. An area health authority (AHA) reported to the regional health authority (RHA) which reported to the Department of Health (DoH). The AHA lasted only a short while and was then abolished in the interests of economy. But the people who were taken on to help the reorganisation have seemed never to disappear. They are resurrected in different jobs again and again and in different places. Some of the senior managers I knew originally entered straight from school and are now grey haired.

The NHS first became obsessed with management in the late 1960s. Sadly, it failed to distinguish between planning and wishing. Wishing does not make it so! Like many other consultants, nurses and everyone else in the NHS, I attended course after course on management. I have a theory that the DoH imported academics from the United States just as their intellectual status was beginning to fade. The shortest lived fad was management by intention. It rapidly became clear that if senior managers, and particularly politicians, declared their intentions there would be no politics. One theory that has not been used is that of Deming* which now controls much of industry. The first law of management should be: "A manager can make it worse". A good manager will, of course, make it better but they are a rare breed.

The changes continue but, for me, they have merged into a blur. The pleasures of working in this district and the lack of serious arguments among colleagues have made medicine a lot easier than dealing with the powers that be. There was little change in the doctors' work until the most recent reorganisation (1991) when I was close to retirement. The nurses suffered from management at all levels, usually with the argument that "they do it in America"! I can see no virtue in replacing Florence Nightingale's ideas with "graduate nurses" who fight with the doctors, leaving the work with patients to be done by the practical nurses.

Some of the reorganisation changes at ward level have been quite batty. When responsibility is more and more closely controlled in all parts of the NHS, why are the junior ward staff called "named nurses" and are accountable but inexperienced and obviously not present 24 hours a day? Several of our local wards are now quietly returning to central authority for the sake of continuity of care.

Costly purchase and sale of buildings

One of the most expensive results of the reorganisation in East Sussex has been the purchase and sale of buildings. Over the years the RHA, née RHB, went from Paddington to East Croydon and then to the largest office block in Bexhill. Built by a building society, it could be compared only with the Transport Workers' Convalescent Home in Eastbourne. With dark glass, bronze window frames, air conditioning, and a very large director's suite on the sixth floor, it was guarded like a fortress. But as far as the local NHS was

---

* Dr W. Edwards Deming holds that the manager and not the worker is responsible for declining levels of quality and productivity.

concerned, the entire staff could have succumbed to a mystery virus and nobody would have noticed for days. The only noticeable thing they did for the local services was to steal all the best secretaries. The senior staff in the RHB were very cross at being rusticated and had little to do with the yokels. The 1991 changes have allowed officers to recivilise in London and as civil servants too!

My worst administrative defeat was over the site of the new hospital, which opened in 1991– some 24 years after the original promise. During the third planning round one potential site was a large open area between Bexhill and Hastings alongside the railway and main coast road. High powered architectural advice decreed the site to be liable to flooding so the NHS refused it. After a decent interval of what seemed like five minutes, the space became a large shopping precinct! The powers that be then decided that the most satisfactory hospital site was at the back of Hastings and, with a planned new road down to the coast, it would have been. Now, the ridge at the back of the town may have been tactically important to the Romans and the Normans but it is only a road between Battle and Rye. The new hospital was completed, the link road to the coast was not, and we still suffer from complications of poor access.

Pleasure of driving to work

All the weird behaviour of the boards and managers cannot take away the sheer spiritual pleasure of driving to work along the seafront and thinking of all my friends in London traffic. The coast has other benefits for doctors. I had to give up water skiing when I bent myself slightly, but just in time the windsurfer was invented. It is the ideal way for the working man to sail: setting up is so fast and sudden immersion in cold water clears the irritations of the day. An additional sybaritic problem to living here is that when the sun shines it takes much moral effort to attend learned meetings.

And the future?

- We have made the NHS too complex and responsible for functions only distantly related to illness.
- Freely treating the sick is a just and reasonable thing for a rich country to do, but the service's sensitivity to political pressure wastes vast amounts of money solving problems that do not exist and failing to solve those that do.
- Surely a board of governors like the BBC would be better than a politically controlled NHS Executive?

Dr Beeching made it hard to reach London so the temptation of country or seaside pursuits is ever present. And if you really do not want to go to that meeting, you can always play golf.

The NHS is the one consumer service which no normal consumer would want a part of unless he or she had to. Demand for therapeutic medicine is clearly not infinite, but political direction has allowed all sorts of duties to be loaded on the service. The motive for most of the reorganisations has been to control costs. Usually, however, the result is higher spending without commensurate clinical benefit. The shortage of funds for direct patient care has been worsened by governments' reluctance to take account of the real level of health service inflation, which in advanced economies is always higher than general inflation.

To control expenditure in the NHS requires control of the number of employees. Those not involved in patient care must show their worth and save their own salary at least, every year. The internal market is artificial and a curious idea for an organisation on a fixed income. It has wasted resources on the negotiations for annual purchaser/provider contracts and, incidentally, has convinced me that many finance officers cannot count. I regret to say it, but I'm glad to be a retired spectator rather than a struggling participant in the NHS. I hope, however, that it will survive to meet the needs of those pensioners like myself who sooner or later may need its care.

24:   Evaluation of health policy: time to rethink

Ray Robinson

Medical practice has traditionally been strongly influenced by biomedical research and by the evaluation of clinical and laboratory procedures. The NHS has comfortably cohabited with and benefited from such research and evaluation and the recent emphasis on the practice of evidence based medicine is a welcome step in this evolving tradition. Paradoxically, despite a decades long trail of financial and organisational change imposed on the NHS, rigorous evaluation of how well the service works and of the effects of new policies has been rare. What was right for medicine was largely ignored in respect of the framework within which "free" comprehensive health care was delivered to the nation.

The reasons for this are legion and stem from the NHS's mixed origins, its size and complexity, constantly changing political priorities, weak management structures, and the powerful influence of clinically motivated doctors in policy making. This lack of evaluation has resulted in wasted resources and less effective preventive and curative care for the community. Rather than rake over the historical whys and wherefores of wasted opportunities, however, I am directing my contribution to the future by examining how we should rethink policy evaluation in the NHS.

Attitudes towards the evaluation of health policy have, however, changed fundamentally over the past six years. When the 1990 NHS reforms were launched, the then Secretary of State, Kenneth Clarke, running true to NHS tradition, had little time for pilot schemes or evaluation. He made it clear that he did not want academics crawling all over the NHS. As a result, no provision was made for formal evaluation of the most radical set of changes ever applied to the NHS system of organisation and finance. Since then official policy has changed dramatically. No policy initiative is now complete without a commitment to evaluation. For those, like me, with a preference for rational policy making, this trend is welcome. What I find less welcome, however, is the apparent absence of understanding about what is possible and appropriate by way of evaluation in complex and rapidly changing policy environments. To appreciate the crux of this dilemma, we need to consider the recent development of the NHS Research and Development (NHS R&D) programme.

Research and development programme

The launch of the NHS R&D programme in 1991 was a major step towards the creation of an evidence base to improve decision making. For the first time, a coherent research infrastructure was put in place which was to be driven by the applied research needs of the service. This commitment to an evidence based approach has subsequently been accompanied by (and contributed towards) a wider set of activities designed to improve clinical performance through the practice of evidence based medicine and the more general pursuit of clinical effectiveness. This desirable trend has had spillover effects in policy areas with the more recent emphasis on evidence based policy. But confusion about what constitutes valid evidence in the latter case poses a problem.

For most medical researchers (whose methodological approach dominates the NHS R&D programme), evaluation means a controlled experiment. The rules of this approach are clear and widely accepted. Following the introduction of an intervention or programme, the research design should control for bias and confounding extraneous factors, so that the impact of the intervention can be isolated and measured. This is the classic approach of laboratory science. Within clinical research, this approach is, of course, pursued through the randomised controlled trial (RCT) which occupies the apex of the accepted hierarchy of evidence.

Sometimes we can extend this approach to non-clinical questions. For example, studies on cost effectiveness and other forms of economic evaluation carried out alongside RCTs often collect information on costs and outcomes in a way that meets the standards of a controlled trial. In most areas of health policy, however, there is far less scope for controlling for factors over which the researcher has little direct influence. In such cases, quasi-experimental methods are often recommended. Probably the most thorough quasi-experiment to be carried out in the health policy area was the health insurance experiment conducted by the RAND Corporation in the United States during the 1970s. This was a randomised trial of over 7700 individuals designed to establish the effects of cost sharing on both the demand for health services and health status. The experiment was a long term one with participants recruited over three years, 1974–1977, and followed for between three and five years. As such, the project was very costly. Even in the USA, with its generous levels of research funding, it is widely recognised that the RAND experiment belongs to the halcyon days of applied social science research and is unlikely to be repeated in the foreseeable future.

Methodological problems in evaluation of policy outcomes

In the UK, those researchers who have sought to use quasi-experimental methods in policy areas have either been restricted to a very narrow set of research questions (for example, the effect of fundholding by general practitioners on hospital referrals or drug prescribing) or have found that the diversity and pace of change affecting the subject under investigation have seriously impeded the approach. The latter considerations are shown quite vividly in the case of the national evaluation of total purchasing, where constant policy change around the 53 first-wave pilot sites has posed formidable problems for the attribution of causality.

Despite these complications, a majority of those funding NHS research and development, and indeed, many researchers themselves, believe that quasi-experimental methods are the only really respectable approach. I see this as posing the very real danger that research will either fail to produce results that meet the funders' expectations and/or be discredited among the policy community because the findings bear little relevance to their needs. What is required is far greater emphasis on the policy world as it is – as opposed to how researchers would ideally like it to be – and the selection of research methods that are appropriate to this world.

If this focus is adopted, other aspects of research design besides those emphasised in controlled experiments become far more important. Let me take the emerging developments in primary care organisation as an example. What is required is formative evaluation with a developmental dimension, an indepth understanding of causality in relation to organisational and individual behaviour, timeliness in the production of evidence, and attention to the cost of evaluation. I will examine these considerations in turn.

In its most general sense, evaluation seeks to define a project, identify its objectives, and assess how far these are met. Objectives may be internal (as defined by the participants) and/or external (as defined by the researchers or other third parties). In many policy areas, however, at the initial stages the nature of the project and its objectives are ill defined. In such cases a formative evaluation which emphasises critical reflection on the process of project design and implementation, as well as the final outcomes, is desirable. This is often described as action research in which the researcher feeds back information to the participants with the aim of assisting the development of the project. Clearly, this process involves a Hawthorne effect and introduces contamination in the controlled experimental sense, but such considerations are of less importance, given the aims of the project.

Turning to the question of causality, I believe there is often a strong case for using in depth qualitative research, alongside quantitative techniques, to gain a fuller understanding of the causes of individual and group behaviour. These causes can assume particular importance when the diverse groups affected by a project or programme have divergent views about its nature and objectives. For example, studies of shifting workload at the primary/ secondary care interface show that different groups have different views about what constitutes a shift and its associated consequences. Their behaviour is governed by these perceptions. Questions such as these are ideally approached through case study investigations, where the aim is to provide a depth of understanding (and possibly to generate hypotheses for subsequent more general testing) about the complex set of factors determining behaviour in ways that large scale trials or surveys cannot achieve.

Several years lead time for quality research

The lead time associated with the completion of a high quality research project can extend over several years. The tasks of research design, sample selection and recruitment, data collection, analysis, and dissemination of results all absorb much time. In contrast, many management and policy decisions have deadlines of months, weeks or even days. For many research projects, this mismatch in timescales is unimportant because they are addressing issues of such fundamental significance that they will remain relevant whatever the short term policy context. This is clearly so with much biomedical research. In many policy areas, however, this is far less likely. For instance, the value of a three year study of fundholding is likely to be questionable if a change of government results in the abolition of the scheme in the second year. If they are seriously interested in informing and influencing the policy process, researchers need to recognise these timescales. Of course, achieving an acceptable balance between the standards expected of rigorous research, and the demanding, short term timetables often set by the users of research findings within the policy community is rarely easy. As a consequence, many researchers are unwilling to compromise and concentrate on longer term projects - though they often continue to berate decision makers for their failure to heed their findings! For others, the task of developing methods of maximum validity and reliability consistent with the policy timescale represents a challenge in its own right.

Evaluation should be cost effective

Finally, there is cost. As in any activity, evaluation should be cost effective. This means that the scale (and cost) of any evaluation project should be proportionate to the expected benefits. If only minor changes, and hence benefits, are expected the cost of the evaluation should reflect this. A good example of this requirement is the pilot schemes expected to be launched as a result of the Primary Care Act 1997. Present indications suggest that there are likely to be several hundreds of these schemes round the country. The Department of Health has stipulated that each must be subject to local evaluation. Many of them, however, are likely to be extremely modest in scope and in my view it would clearly be a waste of resources to undertake elaborate evaluation. In many cases, project monitoring of the type usually associated with accountability, through performance management by health authorities, is likely to be adequate.

Evaluation ...

- aims to define a project, identify its objectives, and assess how far these are met;
- should include qualitative as well as quantitative research;
- is time consuming, with tension between the often long timescale for worthwhile research and the short deadlines of management expectations making an acceptable balance hard to achieve;
- should be cost effective, with the scale and cost of an evaluation project proportionate to the expected benefits;
- requires a far more eclectic approach to its funding that recognises methods other than those of controlled clinical trials.

Taken overall, the argument I have advanced here suggests that other criteria besides those associated with classic controlled experiments need to be given far higher priority in the interests of research that is relevant to policy. There is nothing really new in this argument; indeed, it has been made by numerous researchers over the years. It should not be taken to imply criticism of established scientific methods in either social science or medicine. Rather, it is an argument for the choice of appropriate research methods for the task in hand. Despite its familiarity, however, the message does not seem to have got home as far as much of the NHS R&D programme is concerned. If this programme is genuinely going to address the policy needs of the service in the future, a far more eclectic approach to project funding is required, with due recognition being given to methods other than those of controlled clinical trials. Effective evaluation will contribute to the more efficient use of resources, an important objective when the gap between what patients need and what the community is prepared to afford for a state service grows ever wider.

25:   The changing status of public health: a personal experience

Dame Rosemary Rue

One afternoon in the 1930s, I returned from school in south London to find large jugs of boiled water set aside and all the water taps covered. My mother, anxious and frightened, explained that there was something called typhoid in the water supply and the Medical Officer of Health (MOH) had told her what to do. The front page of the evening paper was filled with his advice. It was serious. An ambulance was in our street and a neighbour was among many who subsequently died. But we could be sure that the MOH knew everything about typhoid and could be trusted to get the outbreak under control. We just had to do exactly as he said. I thought it extraordinary that he had never been to our house, yet knew when it was safe to use the water again. Not long afterwards, he strongly recommended immunisation against diphtheria. Two cousins had died of this disease and a third had survived with his heart affected. Now our family could be protected by the new injections and my parents decided we would be among the first volunteers.

Our non-medical family was, I imagine, fairly typical in its familiarity with infectious disease and in its appreciation of advice from a responsible doctor who was always backed up by our own GP. Public health measures had transformed, within my parents' lifetime, the quality of life in London, the medical profession being respected as much for its preventive approach as for anything it had to offer in the way of treatment. There was a general attitude of collaboration, appearing in the popular press and reinforced in schools, with advice on the improvement of health. The public was given messages about fresh air, sunlight, and diet targeted at tuberculosis, rickets, and anaemia, with admonitions to individuals to take exercise and study First Aid. People, especially poor families, were entreated to consult a doctor if serious symptoms were recognised, without waiting to consider the cost. Persuasion at that time was used by doctors, not patients. There

146

was no hint that medical advice would be other than fully informed and unanimously supported by the profession as a whole. The MOH was a doctor with local standing, a familiar figure with essential public duties. He was the guardian of safety measures for infectious disease control but he also provided basic hospital and community health services. His status derived from his professional qualifications and from half a century of legislation endowing him with powers and responsibilities that were unquestioned. MOHs were chief officers of local authorities which were themselves powerful, stable and mostly well funded.

During the 1939–1945 war years, numerous official health campaigns were aimed at the armed forces and at civilians. Many dealt with infectious disease and could hardly be missed. Food rationing, with its special supplements for expectant mothers and children, surprised everyone by favourably influencing the national diet. The surviving population emerged from its ordeal fitter than ever before. By the time I became a medical student, as the war ended, there was widespread general knowledge of preventive health and a good deal of confidence in the country's ability to maintain and deliver health services, including those of public health.

Public health less of a problem in 1948

As the NHS came into being, concern about the state of the hospitals and the shortage of general practitioners was widespread but public health was thought to be less of a problem. The sanitary infrastructure simply needed repair. Lessons concerning diet and physical fitness, vaccination and immunisation programmes, the logistics of ambulance services and blood supplies had been learned and could be readily applied. Had not the civilian emergency services and the armed forces found ways of solving all the problems using volunteers and minimally trained recruits? If the army could be kept healthy while fighting its way across the world, it would be a simple matter to keep the general population healthy in peacetime. Or so went the argument. The way ahead for ambitious doctors lay in the scientific and technical developments in diagnostic and therapeutic medicine, the new antibiotics, the improved anaesthetics.

At medical school, therefore, public health was out of date, the past, an aspect of medicine best avoided. Such work as was necessary to maintain public health standards set in the Victorian era would be the responsibility of some sort of activity separated from the medical workforce of the future. In this atmosphere, the teaching and examining in the subject failed seriously, at least in the London medical schools. The dull reiteration of historical legislation aroused no interest in a generation of medical students who had been witnessing momentous events almost daily and whose eyes were set on the future horizon. If only there had been some imaginative

147

exercise in topical problem solving and some statistics more recent than the Boer War! I felt vaguely cheated that I qualified without any academic development of my impression that there was a comprehensive, population based aspect to medicine which had positive health goals. But it did not seem that these ideas lay in the province of public health as presented by the medical schools at the time.

Irritating overlaps between public health services and GPs

In the 1950s, with the NHS well established as an organisation of three branches – hospitals, general practice, and public health – my perception as a GP was that the clinical public health services were irritatingly overlapping with my own role. Maternity, child welfare clinics, and school medical examinations were a repeated source of referrals. The need to reassure the patients and respond to local authority doctors who had no therapeutic resources and were not experiencing the same pressures of demand as GPs became irksome. I never met or heard from the MOH

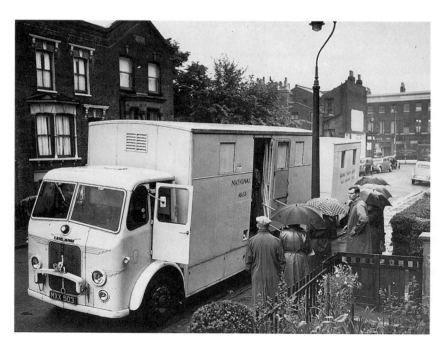

When the NHS was launched many of its buildings were inadequate for the task of providing a comprehensive service. This picture shows a mobile surgery in use in April 1949. Reproduced with permission from Getty Images.

concerning his motives in deploying a medical team apparently to second guess my clinical judgement.

The outcome was abrasive competitiveness between professionals over the health, or more often the sickness, of children and their harassed and confused mothers. I suspect I was at least as tolerant as other GPs in the locality and can see now that there was confusion of roles on both sides, there being no forum for frank communication. Quite unnecessary friction was generated between doctors in public health and general practice. They could have collaborated happily in developing modern primary care. I was grateful at the time for the TB contact and surveillance services but in this field the published papers emanated from specialist chest physicians now in the hospital branch of the NHS. It was developments in the vaccination and immunisation programme – the determined effort to eradicate smallpox, the new triple (diphtheria, pertussis, and tetanus) and Salk polio vaccines – that finally made me recognise the value of the population based medical planning being undertaken by central and local government through the public health branch of the NHS.

By 1960 events drove me halfheartedly into the public health service, where terms and conditions were extremely attractive. The pressures of day to day work were so diminished compared with general practice that I felt both mystified and inadequate. The full-time job occupied about four hours on weekdays, mainly in term time, and I found it possible for short periods to do locum work for singlehanded practices in the vicinity in the remaining 12 hours or so of my accustomed working day. I understood why it was widely considered among doctors that public health was not sharing the workload that the NHS had generated. The impression that public health was a sideline was exacerbated when postgraduate medical education became established (from 1961) and the discipline failed dismally to participate. There were no scheduled academic events, no research training or projects, no publications or conference papers. The annual compilation of the statistics which comprised the report of the MOH led nowhere in terms of medical innovation. There was a waiting time of five years for an uncertain opportunity to join the Diploma of Public Health (DPH) course, which itself looked antiquated, and when I worked out a relevant personal postgraduate programme, I had to resign my post in order to participate.

Eventually, I did achieve a completely unofficial way of providing integrated public health, specialist, and general practitioner services for a small community and discovered how population based medicine could function. The medical profession was by then openly disparaging towards the public health branch of the NHS and it was too late for internal reform. The best route for the future was through the powerful hospital boards. In the Oxford Region, which I joined in 1965, there were imaginative MOHs developing collaborative services with hospital, GPs, and social services and pushing their local authorities into the future.

149

Serious failure to update medical and scientific basis

Unfortunately, the years of isolation, complacency, and relative inactivity, as public health rested on its laurels and failed seriously to update its medical and scientific basis, had condemned its effectiveness as well as its image. The DPH trained doctors had mostly failed as leaders of social services in the face of an explosion of academic progress in that subject and social change in the community. Local authority social services were separated from public health as a preliminary to its integration with academic departments of social medicine and the medical administrative department of regional hospital boards to form the new medical specialty of community medicine.

Community physicians were given a key role in the integrated NHS of 1974. This first reorganisation might have been a simple improvement concerning the delivery of services to a local population but it became submerged in extremely complex and fashionable management arrangements. Doctors from public health had kept abreast of neither medicine nor management and suffered a major defeat in a competitive atmosphere as their local authority power base, together with nearly all their staff and financial resources, disappeared. Some responsibilities within community medicine were allotted to named doctors but most were shared or subject to team management. The official voice which responded to public health anxieties was no longer the familiar MOH who had a permanent commitment to the community but a changing spokesman for an authority or, more alarmingly, a politician. It was confusing for the public and community medicine was a confusing concept for the profession. Meanwhile, general practice was developing rapidly, though still somewhat overwhelmed by hospital and specialist services. Public health became ever less visible, while doctors with old skills and surviving statutory support continued to protect the public's health as best they could in the new context. The numbers who knew how to provide effective health education and surveillance and to control infectious disease were dwindling.

Inevitably, there were some awful incidents which caused public outrage. Two serious outbreaks of communicable disease led to a committee of inquiry into the future of the public health function. The Chief Medical Officer (Donald Acheson) chaired the committee whose report called for the reinstatement of effective control of infection mechanisms and an urgent revision of medical training in the subject. The lost skills and networks were rapidly rediscovered and directors of public health were appointed as officers of authorities with clearly defined responsibilities. The specialty revised its name again to Public Health Medicine, mainly to ensure better understanding of its role by profession and public. The status of the specialty improved, centrally funded recruitment increased, and political support was forthcoming.

Public health issues high on public agenda

During a further decade of NHS upheavals, several highly publicised events have kept public health interests on the political agenda. The demand for prompt, informed advice and accountability for action has risen in connection with new infections, hygiene standards, and the wider areas of health for all. Yet the numbers of doctors entering the specialty are falling again and there is little insistence from the medical profession that an authoritative medical voice is always heard in response to a fresh alarm. While argument persists in the NHS over the costs of training and employing doctors to take public health responsibilities, confusion too often surrounds fresh incidents as politicians, officials, and very specialised experts proclaim their opinions.

Prime points for public health's future

- Public health is and will remain high on the public agenda and its practitioners' status should be commensurate with this.
- A multidisciplinary activity, public health practice must continue to act in a social as well as a medical context.
- Local communities will need a doctor who acts as the GP in public health.
- Valuable skills will be lost unless public health doctors are appropriately educated and funded and supported professionally by colleagues in other specialties.
- The new post of Minister for Public Health is welcome and offers the opportunity for improved co-operation on health matters between government departments.
- Links between national and local levels of public health must be strong and this will depend in large part on the skill of its practitioners and the resources at their disposal.

There is, of course, more to public health than the medical viewpoint. The practice of public health has always been multidisciplinary and has had regard for its social context. No single doctor today could have the comprehensive knowledge expected of the former MOH but information and communication technology can help. A local community needs, as much as it ever did, a doctor who acts as the GP in public health for that population. There seems to be a recurring danger that such support might be lost to a future generation, who would certainly have to retrieve it. Experience indicates that the way to lose public health skills is through failure to educate, fund and maintain professional support for the doctors involved.

The new post of Minister for Public Health could achieve much between government departments and will, I hope, obtain clear advice from the Chief Medical Officer. However, the links have to be strong between national and local levels and their strength depends heavily on the practitioners in the field and their resources. Public health issues are high on the public agenda and likely to remain so. At the end of a switchback century for public health, its status must remain high in the minds of the public and the profession.

26: A student's perspective

James Stoddart

I was born in an NHS hospital in Scotland, on New Year's Day, 1975. It was my proverbial cradle. I've been brought up with a NHS and became a medical student under the NHS. Even though I am a "Thatcher's child" and there were difficult times for the health service over the 1980s, the NHS is still here. In August 1998, one month after the 50th anniversary, I hope to start my first house job and I expect to spend most of my working life with the NHS. The Welfare State – with the health service as monarch – is meant to be there for us from the cradle to the grave. When I "hit" the grave will there still be a NHS and what form will it take?

This is an essay (in the loosest sense of the word) on the "student's perspective" of the health service. What does the NHS mean to students? What does it do for us and what do we (if anything) do for it? We are students at university medical schools but without the NHS – its hospitals and family practitioner and public health services – where would we see our patients and from whom would we learn? Also, how do the NHS and the medical schools work together? I and my contemporaries are students at a time of change. To give readers a perspective on my short time in the NHS as a student and some thoughts on the service's future, what better way than to see how it affects my daily routine?

8.30 am: professorial ward round

This ward round is to be missed on pain of death. When I heard that I was on the Prof's firm I had mixed emotions. Early on in one's career it is a struggle to get to grips with the "relationship" between universities and the NHS. The doctors on the Prof's firm are all honorary consultants and seem just to do lots of research: did they ever do a medical degree, are they proper doctors? We see endless patients with random, double barrelled syndrome number 37 – his particular field of research – but less of the routine stuff than do friends on the common or garden NHS firms. So, after being grilled on said esoteric syndromes, the ward round finishes and I walk to

153

outpatients, musing that luckily the professor writes a good chapter in the textbook on his superspecialty.

9.30 am: outpatients

Outpatients are seen in the old wing of the hospital. Walking along the sparkling corridors of the 1970s block, I wonder why it is that modern buildings are very functional inside but very ugly on the outside while older buildings are quite hopeless inside but attractive to look at. Pre-NHS hospital architecture is on the whole impressive but depressingly inadequate inside. As I walk down the corridor I am reminded that it rained last night by the line of buckets marking the way.

The first patient needs a simple operation. The consultant asks her the million dollar question (quite literally), "Is your GP a fundholder?". Luckily, the patient's GP is a fundholder and she can have her operation within a couple of months. The next patient is not so lucky: her GP is not a fundholder, so she has to wait for the next financial year for surgery as the health authority has run out of money. Even as a medical student this strikes one as unfair and I (politely) rant to the consultant who agrees with me, but can't do anything about it. Later, I ask my consultant if I may be excused to go to theatre to watch a particular procedure the registrar is doing – a practical part of my education. "Oh, all elective lists have had to be cancelled this week – sorry. Too many emergencies!". Funding of the NHS raises its ugly rear again. The patient misses his operation: I miss my education. If lists are being cancelled, on whom am I going to be taught? Also, what happens if my week with the ear, nose and throat department next year clashes with a bad financial week for the health authority? No elective ENT lists, no ENT patients, and no ENT clinical teaching. Obviously, the NHS cuts are adversely affecting patients' well-being, but they are also affecting our education. This "business-run" NHS is not investing in its assets for the future. I get annoyed and decide it's time for lunch.

12 midday: lunch

We have lunch in the opted out, privately run, open-to-tender canteen. A new, chalked sign on a piece of blackboard announces that HospFast has recently won the tender to provide all the food at the hospital. I walk hungrily to the displays of food. The "food attendants" do look different from the last lot. Dave, my personal "food attendant", wears a blue striped shirt and matching bow tie and a straw hat with a blue band around the rim. The last lot had plain red shirts, white bow ties and no hats. Chicken curry with rice please, I ask. Said foodstuff is slopped onto my tray...with a smile. At the till, Jean gives me a leaflet explaining HospFast's goal and ten stage plan. Interestingly, nothing is mentioned of trying to make the food taste better (it tastes foul – no pun intended) or make it cheaper (it costs more). The NHS/trusts/hospital, whatever they are, get a new company every year to provide the same food, at a higher price, served up by the same people wearing a different uniform and getting lower wages. Who is happy? I don't think Dave and Jean are and certainly I'm not. But the trust is and that, of course, is all that matters.

2.00 pm: afternoon "on take"

I am on "on take" – that is, helping to admit emergency patients. After finishing lunch I am promptly bleeped down to casualty, where an "acute abdomen" is waiting for me. (How easy it is to slip into depersonalising jargon about our patients.) I will clerk the patient's present history and clinical details and present these to the Senior House Officer who will ridicule me. The SHO will then present his version to the registrar and as that doctor has just passed the specialist fellowship exams, the SHO is ridiculed in turn. I am speedily discovering that medicine is just a game and as a student you are just learning the hierarchical rules so that in time you can play too! I finally track down a nurse – they do all seem to be extraordinarily busy – and ask where the patient is. "In the sun lounge: bed 3." The sun lounge is the euphemism used in my hospital for the corridor. All the ward beds are full, so new patients wait in the sun lounge. At least the patient is near the door and is getting some light.

But, hold on, this is all wrong. Why are patients waiting in the corridor? When consultants wax lyrical about their time on the house and the interesting japes they got up to, the examination in corridors of patients who have been waiting for a doctor for several hours never features in the anecdote. What never ceases to amaze me is that the patients seem happy enough with their lot. Even though this man is in a lot of pain, he doesn't seem to mind the long wait in the corridor. To him, all doctors are superb and he congratulates me for wanting to become a doctor and so on and so forth. The public still love the NHS despite its many problems. I eventually finish my "on take" duties and leave the very stressed house officers behind, contemplating, with a frisson of alarm, that a year hence that overstressed house officer will be me.

Back home: thoughts on the NHS

Back home, I ponder what it will really be like as a house officer, senior house officer, Calman specialist registrar and finally as a consultant. My brief career in medicine as a student is affected by the NHS and it is all too easy to be negative about the health service. A relaxing cup of coffee calms my emotions and I realise that all is not doom and gloom in the NHS! The public still has a lot of respect for "their" health service and for the people who work in it. The interest people show when I say I am a medical student is heartening. Furthermore, we can see how dear to people's hearts the NHS is when election time comes. Who is doing what to the NHS through whom is closely and publicly scrutinised, ranking highly with personal taxation (a strange bedfellow indeed) as a vote winner or loser.

The NHS remains free at the point of delivery and access is according to need: these are still its major "selling" points, to use marketing terminology. We, as a nation, are proud of it and comparisons are regularly made with other health care systems in the world, particularly the USA, in which health care provision is not so universal. At least, when I am a doctor I hope that one of my routine questions to patients will not have to be "How do you mean to pay for your health care?". I am optimistic and it is reassuring that when we are ill huge health care resources await if needed: they are only, potentially, a phone call to the GP away.

The future

I believe that:

- Britain's health care system will still be called the NHS when I retire;
- the NHS will change—21st century medicine will be quite different from 1948 and 1998;
- one compelling reason for survival of the service is that politicians know it would be electoral suicide to dismantle it;
- the NHS will be based on different principles from those underlying the Beveridge report of the 1940s;
- people will have to realise that new technologies and rising demands will require more resources;
- whether by extra taxation or other means, those resources will have to be found – a brutal truth behind the rumours (circulating as I write) of the newly elected Labour Government "thinking the unthinkable" on introducing GP visiting and hospital hotel charges;
- student teaching will have to be focused on people and patients in the community;
- students must learn about health politics and management.

Student teaching must change

The way the NHS is used to teach students will have to change. Until the past decade some people stayed in hospital for many days or even weeks. The spin-off for students was that they had plenty of hands on, clinical experience. Now some patients are in for less than a day and the student is losing out on "teaching material", if patients will forgive the description. The solution seems clear. If patients are spending more time being unwell in the community than in hospitals, students should also spend more time in the community learning from patients there. To an extent, this has already started in some medical schools. Cambridge, for example, now has a GP based clinical course. But this will have to become the norm in every medical school. The NHS should still help in teaching students in the hospital setting, but this has to be complementary to teaching in the community.

The medical student curriculum is under severe pressure. Even so, I believe it to be vital for the doctors of tomorrow's NHS that they can develop informed opinions on the service. So medical courses really should have a forum for debating health politics. This might be in a formal lecture setting or as informal group tutorials. Students and doctors need information to make judgements. Ill informed or emotional kneejerk reactions to events are unhelpful to the NHS and the medical profession. Though as a student I see the good and bad points of the NHS, I cannot do a lot about them. This will change, I hope, when I finally qualify (fingers crossed) in August 1998. As a doctor, I will work for our National Health Service well into the next century and sincerely hope to see its centenary in 2048, when I will be a retired but sprightly 73 year old.

27: A professor of therapeutics looks back

Owen Wade

Just after the war I was a young doctor working in London. If I went home for a weekend, I travelled from Paddington on a Friday evening, when Welsh MPs were returning to their constituencies. If George Hall, our local MP, saw me, he would invite me into his compartment (first class). Often his companion was Aneurin Bevan, Minister of Health in Attlee's Cabinet, and they would hold long and interesting discussions about the development of a national health service.

Bevan had been subjected to virulent and unpleasant press criticism and I recall how impressed I was to find this supposed ogre an intelligent, well balanced, well informed, and interesting man. I thought, then, how it was all too easy for the press to misrepresent a man's character. I think now, as then, that whereas we need a free press, it should act responsibly.

To my mind the great early achievement of the NHS was that it became possible to employ a high standard of consultant staff in hospitals throughout our country. Until then, in many areas where there was little private practice-for instance, South Wales-it had been difficult for consultants to make a reasonable living.

Perhaps even more important, however, were the pioneering efforts of family doctors like Ronald Gibson (Hampshire), Ekke Kuensberg (Edinburgh), and Donald Crombie (Birmingham) in developing group practices. The recommendation made by the BMA, led by Solly Wand, a Birmingham GP and its Council's chairman, that part of the Danckwerts award (meant to supplement GPs' salaries) should be used instead to fund group practices was a remarkably far sighted and generous decision. Now almost forgotten in the mists of time, it allowed nurses and other professionals to be recruited to these practices. The result in the 1960s – boosted by the founding of the Royal College of General Practitioners and agreement on the Family Doctors' Charter – was a marked improvement in primary health care and the near elimination of the isolated singlehanded practitioner – surely the greatest achievement of the NHS.

Another valuable feature of those early days was that junior clinical staff could move easily between posts in the NHS, the universities, and the Medical Research Council (MRC) without any financial or pensions problems. I know because I worked for all three in succession! Let me fulfil my task of reviewing the NHS by briefly highlighting some key events in its 50 year history.

Preventive medicine

During the war a successful programme of immunisation of children against diphtheria had been carried out. One of the early achievements of the NHS was the introduction of a much more comprehensive immunisation programme.

The standing of the medical officers of health in those days was high and their contribution to preventive medicine was enormous. My uncle was the Chief Medical Officer of Wales and he and my father discussed these developments with enthusiasm. (Dame Rosemary Rue discusses the fate of public health in Chapter 25–ED.).

Streptomycin: groundbreaking controlled clinical trials

Those early days of the NHS were exciting. To those of us who had seen patients dying of streptococcal and staphylococcal infections, of diphtheria, gas gangrene or subacute bacterial endocarditis, penicillin seemed like magic. The great disappointment was that it had no effect on the tubercle bacillus *Mycobacterium tuberculosis*.

Then in 1948 streptomycin arrived. The MRC, with the guidance of Geoffrey Marshall and Austin Bradford Hill, decided that the limited supply available would best be employed in a rigorously planned "controlled clinical trial". Patients aged 15–30 with bacteriologically proved acute progressive bilateral pulmonary tuberculosis of recent origin were admitted to the first trial. Assessment of the progress of each patient was based on X-ray pictures, weight, temperature, erythrocyte sedimentation rate, and bacillary content of the sputum. It was made by an independent panel of a clinician and two radiologists who had played no part in the treatment of the patients and did not know which patients were receiving streptomycin.

At the end of six months of treatment, four of the 55 streptomycin treated patients had died; while 14 of the 52 patients who had not received streptomycin had died. But streptomycin given alone had its problems. Toxic damage to the auditory and vestibular (balance) systems had been anticipated, but the rapid development of resistance to streptomycin by the tubercle bacillus had not. When another drug, para-aminosalicylic acid (PAS), effective against the tubercle bacillus, was discovered, two further trials using combinations of PAS and streptomycin were carried out. These were planned so that there was no need to include another control group of patients who received neither drug.

This was a wonderful and groundbreaking piece of work. The comprehensive planning and analysis of these three relatively small controlled clinical trials became a model for the assessment of new drugs. Bradford Hill and Archie Cochrane, with whom I was privileged to work in Cardiff, influenced medical practice in Britain profoundly. Many years later, when I visited the American Food and Drugs Administration in Washington, the British practice of accepting as proof of a new drug's efficacy only the results of properly conducted and properly "controlled" clinical trials was spoken of with awe and envy.

Anaesthesia

When I was a student ether and chloroform were still being widely used by the open drop technique. I gave many anaesthetics by this method for my father. In order to obtain relaxation of the abdominal muscles, so essential for intra-abdominal surgery, the patient had to be given such a big concentration of anaesthetic that paralysis of the medulla and respiratory arrest was always a threatening danger. This was to change dramatically when curare and other muscle relaxants became available and the anaesthetic agents were needed only in low concentrations to render the patient unconscious. At the same time anaesthetic equipment was vastly improved by manufacturers, and a new cadre of specialist anaesthetists appeared, and a superb training programme for young anaesthetists was created, with major contributions from Mackintosh at Oxford and Mushin at Cardiff.

Thalidomide: a landmark disaster

In the 1950s, we were well aware of the occasional occurrence of adverse reactions to sulphonamides, streptomycin, corticosteroids and, more rarely, penicillin. Though these might be serious and sometimes fatal, such were the benefits derived from these drugs that these reactions were acceptable.

It was at a congress of gynaecologists at Kiel in October 1961 that attention was first drawn to the increasing prevalence of children born with limb deformities (phocomelia) and at a meeting of paediatricians in Düsseldorf on 19 November, Dr Lenz first suggested that Contergan, a proprietary sedative containing thalidomide taken by mothers during pregnancy, might be the cause.

In Britain, there were at least 500 live births of children with phocomelia, some dreadfully disabled. This disaster left its mark not only on the children but on the medical profession, the pharmaceutical industry, and the public. It led in this country to the creation of the Committee on Safety of Drugs

(CSD), with Derrick Dunlop as its chairman, and later to the statutory Medicine Commission and the Committee on Safety of Medicines.

Legal proceedings against Distillers Ltd, who had marketed thalidomide in Britain, ground on slowly but never reached a court of law. Instead, the company was arraigned, judged, and found guilty by the *Sunday Times* and damages were paid to the parents of the children who had suffered. This assuaged the conscience of a public appalled at the slowness of the legal proceedings.

It would have been far better, however, had the case gone promptly to a court and both sides of the case been heard. In the light of the knowledge, or rather the lack of knowledge, about drug actions that existed in 1961, I doubt whether the company would have been found guilty of negligence. It would perhaps have become clearer how unfair it is at present that enormous payments are made to the relatively few children born with mental or physical defects where negligence can be proved, while the help given to the majority of children born with congenital defects, when there has been no negligence and no drugs can be blamed, is by comparison derisory.

Adverse reactions to oral contraceptives

One of the first actions of the CSD was to institute a system for doctors to report their suspicions about patients' adverse reactions to drugs. Several reports of thromboembolic complications in women taking oral contraceptives were received and a warning was issued in 1967. By 1969, Bill Inman, Medical Officer of the Adverse Reaction Subcommittee of the CSD, was able to show that these complications, though rare, were more common in patients taking contraceptives with high oestrogen content.

It was agreed that all doctors should be informed of this finding before any public announcement was made. But owing to factors outside the control of the CSD the information was presented to the public prematurely in dramatic and unsuitable terms by the media. Totally unnecessary public anxiety was created so that thousands of women descended on their family doctors who had not yet received the CSD letter. Such media generated public anxiety about various treatments has, unfortunately, occurred on several subsequent occasions.

Drug utilisation research

There was another very unexpected consequence of the thalidomide disaster. In Northern Ireland, prescriptions written by doctors went to the Northern Ireland General Health Services Board, where the details of every prescription were transferred to Hollerith sorting cards (after 1964 to a computer) so that pharmacists could be paid promptly. In January 1962 my

161

colleague, Peter Elmes, suggested that if the cards for 1961 were still available we would be able to trace every woman who had been prescribed thalidomide.

Unfortunately, in those days, as soon as pharmacists were paid, the records were destroyed. From then on, however, with the help of Dr Hunter, Medical Officer of the Health Services Board, we were able to undertake detailed research on the prescribing of all doctors in Northern Ireland. In 1969, with the help of the World Health Organisation, this work was extended first to Norway and Sweden and later to other European countries.

These studies show fascinating differences in prescribing within each country and even greater differences in prescribing between countries. It has become clear that the prescribing of drugs, which we had naively assumed to have been done solely on a rational basis, is profoundly influenced by tradition, doctors' concepts of disease, patients' expectations of treatment, the marketing and advertising of drug companies, the misconceptions of the media and the health service policies concerning the reimbursement of the cost of prescription charges. Each of these may vary greatly from country to country.

Cancer therapy and immune suppression

Strangely, it was the observation during the 1914–1918 war, among the survivors of those exposed to mustard gas, that the rapidly dividing white cell precursors in the bone marrow were depressed that was to lead in the 1950s to the first development of cytotoxic drugs like busulphan, mercaptopurine, and cyclophosphamide. These were used to treat leukaemia and Hodgkin's disease.

Since then the strategy of using in combination two or more cytotoxic drugs of differing action in interfering with cell division and mitosis has been encouraging. Alkylating agents like cyclophosphamide, antimetabolites like methotrexate, cytotoxic antibiotics like doxorubicin, the plant vinca alkaloids, sex hormones and sex hormone antagonists like tamoxifen occasionally cure but more frequently palliate. It is a tribute to the skill of the modern oncologist that a balance is so often obtained between effective anticancer cell therapy and damage to the normal cells. I have to admit, however, that the treatment of many cancers – breast, stomach, and pancreas, for example – is still most disappointing.

Interestingly, the development of related immunosuppressive drugs like cyclosporin, mycophenolate, mofetil, and azothioprin has allowed the improvement of transplant surgery of the kidney, liver, and heart. This has enabled previously doomed patients to live longer and in reasonable health.

Indeed, people are generally living longer in industrially advanced societies. This is due not only to better housing, hygiene, and diets than those of their 19th century predecessors, but also to modern medical care. Even so, we must never forget that for the aged, though treatment may postpone it, death is inevitable. We must always strive to ensure that dying and death are as peaceful and as dignified as possible. That can be achieved only by the very highest standards of medical and nursing care. I commend to our government a careful examination of the way in which the social services and the medical services of Northern Ireland were successfully amalgamated in 1948. It made the care of the elderly and infirm much easier and more flexible and efficient than I was to find it when I returned to England in 1971.

Thoughts on the future

In Third World countries high mortality and high morbidity will remain a major problem. What they need most is money not medicines – money means better water, better food, better hygiene, and good primary health care. And as health improves, population control will become more important. What is needed is a safe, cheap, single annual dose, oral contraceptive.

In the wealthy countries of Europe and the Pacific rim, financial resources are never going to be sufficient to do all that is possible for every patient. Decisions will be difficult as populations age, people's expectations rise, and medicine advances.

When the young doctor of today retires, he or she will have seen:

- more effective drugs for the treatment of viral diseases;
- better therapy for malaria;
- new drugs for neoplastic disease;
- methods of altering the genetic code to eliminate many congenital diseases;
- a plethora of drugs of little real value marketed by the aggressive multinational drug companies of the future;
- extensive information – but not necessarily wisdom – available on the electronic "network".

28:   The NHS and medical research: uncertainty and excitement

Sir David Weatherall

For those of us who qualified in the 1950s, the existence of the NHS was taken for granted. We had never known any other system of medical care. Our teaching hospitals seemed to run smoothly under the benign administration of a superintendent and matron backed up by a board of governors and if there were financial or managerial problems, they never seemed to percolate through to students or junior medical staff. As we broke our teeth on our first clinical research projects, grants were relatively easy to obtain and nobody ever questioned our right to make use of the facilities of our hospitals and their laboratories for our studies.

In those days it was customary for a budding young academic clinician to travel to the USA as part of his or her education. There, though clinical and research facilities were often of a standard which we had never dreamed possible and some aspects of clinical practice and science were many years ahead of the United Kingdom, we entered a completely new world for the provision of patient care. Personal health insurance was mandatory, every examination and investigation had to be costed, and though the quality of medical practice was remarkably advanced, we had the uneasy feeling that it was not evenly spread throughout the population.

As we sat in our well appointed clinics, we saw families literally ruined by the cost of a serious illness. Furthermore, it was more difficult to carry out the kind of clinical research which requires the collection of large numbers of patients with a particular disease; co-operation between hospitals and between hospitals and the community was not nearly as effective as in the NHS. I suspect that many of us, though heavily tempted to remain in the USA, returned home mainly because we pined for the NHS. I have to admit, however, that in my case the reassuring voice of John Arlott on the BBC's Third Programme, not to mention the pleasures of an English pub lunch, also figured high in the decision making process!

I have no doubt that the NHS has played a major role in any success in

164

biomedical research that this country has achieved over the past 50 years. The provision of health care under a single government agency has made it possible to carry out large scale epidemiological studies with greater efficiency. The "knock for knock" arrangement, whereby university physicians and surgeons offered clinical services to their teaching hospitals while the latter, in return, provided clinical and laboratory facilities for teaching and research at the bedside and in the clinic, worked extremely well for many years. And the close interaction between hospitals and between general practitioners and the hospital services across the country allowed research workers to collect large numbers of patients with particular diseases that interested them. Observational clinical research became an integral part of the life of most British teaching centres.

NHS environment facilitates research

Against this background of co-operation the environment created by the NHS was a central player in the particularly successful period for the development of the biomedical sciences in the UK in the 1960s and 1970s. The spawning of clinical epidemiology and the institution of long term observational studies in the community, together with the multicentre trials and a very high quality of whole patient physiological research at the bedside, allowed the UK to achieve internationally competitive standards of clinical investigation, at least in some centres, during this period. A few examples must suffice. Many important epidemiological investigations were carried out, notably the long term follow-up observations on smokers which led to the recognition of the unequivocal relationship between smoking and lung cancer and heart disease. Following the classic study of the use of multiple drugs for the treatment of tuberculosis, the Medical Research Council trials of the management of childhood leukaemia started to make major inroads into improving the prognosis of this distressing disease and some progress was at last made in the control of different forms of adult leukaemia and lymphoma. Initially by the study of volunteers and later by trials involving different centres, methods were developed to prevent rhesus haemolytic disease of the newborn. Excellent clinical research was carried out in NHS teaching hospitals, which underpinned such developments as transplant surgery, the flowering of clinical genetics and immunology, and improvements in diagnosis and management which touched on every clinical specialty.

It was during this period, and in no small part because of NHS facilities and the availability of good record linkage programmes, that clinical epidemiology began to play a major part in changing the emphasis of medical practice from treatment to prevention. The concept of "risk factors" started to evolve and it became evident that many of the important killers of middle and old age might be preventable, at least to some extent.

This was a remarkable change in medical thinking. Diseases like myocardial infarction, stroke, and cancer, previously lumped together as "degenerative disorders" and by inference the inevitable price to be paid for growing old, now began to be seen as the result of years of exposure to tobacco, rich food, lack of exercise, and other bad habits which made life tolerable. There is no doubt that for both community research and clinical investigation at the bedside, the 1960s and 1970s were a period of major achievement, much of which relied heavily on the NHS.

NHS changes affect research

Following the first major reorganisation of the health services, with the disbandment of the boards of governors and the creation of regional and area health authorities, the excellent research environment created by the NHS could no longer be taken for granted. Several factors combined about this time to place pressures on academic medicine which it had not previously encountered. With the loss of the boards of governors, medical schools now had to negotiate with tiers of NHS authorities. Pressures on hospitals increased, with greater clinical and administrative workloads, and medical academics found themselves with less time to pursue research. In the early 1980s government funding for both the universities and research councils became much tighter and medical schools felt under siege.

However, after the NHS had settled down again, it came to the rescue. As university staff were lost owing to cuts in government funding and it became impossible to create new posts to pursue some of the exciting areas of medical research and practice that were evolving, regional health authorities often stepped in and provided academic posts for the universities. This forward looking action by the NHS enabled them not only to survive but even to expand their activities during this difficult period and could be counted extremely successful. It helped medical schools to maintain and develop their teaching and research, while simultaneously enabling the NHS to attract a very high calibre of clinicians who were able to develop new areas of patient care. Thus despite the major reorganisations and increased bureaucracy in the NHS during this period, the service managed to remain an excellent vehicle for clinical research and epidemiological studies. Many medical schools owed their continued existence, both for teaching and research, to the NHS's support.

During the latter half of the 1980s and early 1990s, several changes took place in both the pattern of medical research and the organisation of the NHS. These, together with a further reduction of funding for the universities, conspired to produce a particularly difficult time for biomedical research in Britain. Following the revolution in biology of the post-DNA era, there was a change of emphasis from the study of patients and their organs to the analysis of pathology at the level of molecules and cells. While this offered remarkable possibilities for improving our understanding of the mechanisms of disease and, in the longer term, for the development of more humane and effective methods of treatment, most medical schools in the UK had neither the facilities nor staff to take advantage of these new advances. Meanwhile, the clinical and administrative workload of the NHS continued to increase and medical schools were trying to carry out epidemiological and clinical research, as before, and to take on the added load of these new and highly sophisticated approaches to the investigation of disease.

NHS upheavals put great pressure on academics

As these changes in the pattern and scope of biomedical research were beginning to bite, the NHS found itself in the throes of a further series of extensive reorganisations. The first was the 1984 introduction of the Griffiths proposals on general management at all levels in hospitals, regions, and districts. Before the dust had settled on that radical change came yet another complete upheaval of the health services. The purchaser/provider split and the teaching hospitals' change of status to independent trusts, rapidly made the NHS unrecognisable as the institution we had worked in during the 1950s and 1960s. It was, in effect, transformed into an industry, complete with new tiers of managers, many of whom knew nothing about clinical practice, not to mention research and teaching.

Academic medicine came under enormous pressures in the 1990s. Clinical academics, together with their NHS colleagues, spent hours on committees trying to make the new organisation work and, to add to their problems, the "knock for knock" arrangements which had served academic medicine so well in the past had to be taken apart. The service increment for teaching (SIFT) with its research component, a longstanding arrangement that recognised the costs of teaching and research, had to be dissected in detail and completely new approaches to the costing of teaching and research in the university hospitals had to be understood and implemented. In addition, both the hospital services and the universities were becoming increasingly underfunded for the work that was expected of them. The morale of clinical academics reached its lowest ebb since the NHS was created.

I have no doubt that the 1991 reorganisation of the NHS has had a deleterious effect on many aspects of clinical research, a problem which was highlighted by the relatively poor performance by many British medical schools in the government's most recent research assessment exercise. The time required on committees helping NHS colleagues to make sense of the endless reforms and quests for efficiency, the dissolution of the "knock for knock" arrangements, demands for a radical new approach to postgraduate training following the Calman report on specialist training, and an ever increasing clinical load left even less time for research. To add to these problems, the General Medical Council (GMC) decided that this was a good time to press for major changes in the pattern of training for medical students.

Internal market disrupts epidemiological studies

It was a rude awakening when, after following groups of patients for many years from different parts of the country for invaluable observational studies of the natural history of disease, letters would appear from administrators in other regions saying that they were unwilling to bear the costs of referring patients across boundaries because they could be looked after quite adequately closer to home. Not only did this reduce the effectiveness of this type of research but it had a very distressing effect on patients with chronic diseases, many of whom had been looked after by one centre for many years and now found that they were not allowed to visit it again. In addition, it became more difficult to carry out drug trials and some of the major pharmaceutical companies in the UK began to find it easier to test their products in the USA, a situation which would not have occurred in the NHS of even ten years ago. Many trusts were unable or unwilling to pay for drugs for clinical trials; cancer research was hit particularly hard.

The appointment of a director of research and development for the NHS, backed up by a series of regional directors, led to the establishment of a few excellent health service research centres and to a much more critical approach to how the NHS spends its relatively small amount of research and development funds. Unfortunately, however, this exercise did not free any new funding for research. Furthermore, it is not yet clear whether the newly developed programmes based on the Culyer report for the local management of this type of research, which have a distinctly bureaucratic feel about them, will further the research potential of the NHS.

It would be unfair to place all the responsibility for the current concerns over the future of biomedical research in Britain on the shortcomings of those who run the NHS. Both the staffing levels and research facilities of our university teaching centres have fallen behind those required for many of them to hope to be internationally competitive. Furthermore, productive research has not been helped by the combination of the rigid training expectations of the royal colleges. Together with uncertainties about whether, under the new career development programmes introduced by the Calman report, I am doubtful whether our most talented young people will be able to find the time to spend the periods of research training and uncluttered thinking that is so vital if they are to develop their talents.

These problems however, are largely organisational, and should be solvable. Much more worrying are the increasing pressures from the GMC

168

and Department of Health to reduce the scientific emphasis of medical education in the belief that this will produce a generation of more caring, socially adaptable, and efficient doctors. If pressed too far, this substantial shift in the emphasis of medical education could do serious harm to our next generation of medical scientists. The basic biological sciences have enormous potential for patient care. Provided that these are taught in this context and balanced by an equal emphasis on the ethical, pastoral, and communication skills of good doctoring, there is no reason why they should not retain their vital role in the education of doctors of the future.

An exciting future for research

Many exciting developments are in the offing.

- The Medical Research Council has interesting new ideas for the reorganisation of biomedical research funding.
- The Wellcome Trust, in collaboration with the NHS and hospital trusts, is planning to establish several clinical research centres in the UK which should provide badly needed facilities in which to carry out investigations on patients.
- The rise of molecular medicine, and its future partnership with epidemiology, offers the possibility of major advances in preventive medicine in the future.
- The molecular approach to the study of disease is also forging closer associations between medical schools and the pharmaceutical industry to ensure the most rapid and effective outcome of new knowledge about disease for its application to patient care.
- Hitherto undreamed of advances in the management of cancer, genetic disease, and the refractory diseases of middle and old age are on the horizon, all of which will require a partnership between universities, industry, and the NHS if they are to move rapidly into the clinic.
- Equally exciting prospects for health service research are on the horizon, with the advent of new information technology and the generation of more critical approaches to the provision of preventive medicine and clinical care.

The past 12 years have seen constant upheavals in the NHS owing to one major reorganisation after another. If it is left alone for a while and allowed to settle down, there is no reason why it should not resume its place as the best environment in the world in which to carry out clinical research. If the government wishes to improve services to patients, it should at least test new measures by properly designed pilot studies rather than indulge in the kind of massive, overnight reorganisations that have been the pattern of previous reforms; the NHS cannot go on suffering as a political pawn.

Clearly, as the NHS celebrates its 50th birthday its future as a vehicle for medical research looks less certain than at any time since it was established. At the same time, there are many other factors that threaten the future of young medical scientists. However, birthdays, as well as times for taking stock of the past and present, should be occasions for celebration and looking to the future with optimism. And on this occasion there is still much about which to be optimistic. Medical research has the potential to move into the most exciting phase of its development and one in which the NHS, if it is allowed to continue in the spirit of its founders, can and must play a major role.

29: The pharmaceutical industry: clinical saviour or commercial villain?

Frank Wells

Nothing was further from my mind when I became a medical student not quite 50 years ago, than that I would finish my professional employment in the pharmaceutical industry. Though I had initial doubts about moving into commerce, I found a stimulating professional environment. I count myself privileged to have been part of it.

Fifty years ago we had penicillin, antacids, digoxin, reserpine, tar, and radiotherapy. We still have them, but we also have cephalosporins, H_2 antagonists, ACE inhibitors, beta-blockers, corticosteroids, and chemotherapy. My second list is not necessarily either the latest available in the fields of infection, peptic ulceration, heart failure, hypertension, dermatoses or cancer or by any means "the best", because superlatives are forbidden in the pharmaceutical industry for fear of breaching The Code, let alone the advertising regulations. But these lists show without any effort on my part (for they were the first treatments and alternatives which came into my head) that there has been significant change for the better over the past 50 years in the availability of effective medicines.

What has the NHS achieved over the past five decades which has itself influenced the pharmaceutical industry? At the very least, it has provided an enviable degree of stability in providing health care to the nation, something of great value in the research context. Where else in the world is the entire population able to register with their own general practitioners, who maintain a complete record of their patients' medical histories from the cradle to the grave? It is hardly surprising, therefore, that the international pharmaceutical industry is much attracted to invest in research in the United Kingdom, despite the vicissitudes inflicted on the NHS by various governments, because of the ready availability of easily identifiable patient subjects in virtually any given category of disease.

Willingness to invest

This willingness to invest in research has been paralleled by developments in setting standards, largely led by UK initiatives. We are proud, too, of our Faculty of Pharmaceutical Medicine, for example, which is unique in the world in providing a higher academic qualification for doctors wishing to become pharmaceutical physicians.

Standards impress me. Call them guidelines, rules, a code of practice or what you will, by hook or by crook the pharmaceutical industry operates to high standards. It does so both when the standards are set as regulatory requirements or when they are adopted voluntarily and that in itself is greatly reassuring. But I realise that very few people outside the industry understand or even know about these standards. Maybe they take them for granted, but most people probably do not think about such things.

Good clinical research practice (GCP) standards were founded in the UK. Undoubtedly this was in part a result of a stable NHS, a ready source of patient subjects, a pool of motivated investigators, and a determination within the UK based industry to set high standards. GCP is now an intentionally harmonised concept. As well as GCP guidelines there are good laboratory practice (GLP) guidelines – inherently part of the research process – and good manufacturing practice (GMP) guidelines, these referring to the quality of finished products. All these are strengthened by the presence of a regulatory authority inspectorate.

That the pharmaceutical industry here has been successful in setting standards for the clinical research process has been clearly shown by requests made to it by representatives of academia to advise on the setting of similar standards for research that is not industry sponsored. The response from clinical academic bodies has been positive.

University research workers were aware of the danger of being seen to have less stringent standards in academic research than those applying to industry sponsored research. This was as important a contribution towards the science of healing as the successful introduction of newer and better medicines.

Fraud in research

I cannot resist a reference to fraud in clinical research, as in my capacity as Medical Director of the Association of British Pharmaceutical Industry I have spent more time tackling it than on anything else. I can do so because the UK industry has comprehensively adopted a forthright policy of taking appropriate action against any doctor generating false data with an intent to deceive. This is tough standard setting, for which the industry must take credit. Nor can I resist a reference to information aimed at the prescriber, the dispenser and above all the patient. Here, too, the industry has done its level best, though maybe it has not been quite as successful as it has been elsewhere.

These statements sound like industry propaganda. Do I believe them? Yes, I do. I have met so many committed and dedicated individuals in the industry during my decade working for it that I am convinced that they not only want to achieve high standards in all they do, but that they also succeed in doing so far more often than not. Additionally, however, the industry is highly regulated and has to stick to tough rules, though sometimes the industry's self-imposed rules – at least in the UK – are even tougher than the law. This applies in advertising, where the Prescription Medicines Code of Practice Authority is recognised as being the strictest self-regulatory body in the world. Its existence minimises the chances of prosecution under the advertising regulations of the Medicines Act.

Success stories in the commercial world which are compatible with improvements in the quality of life are few and far between. Here, however, we have the commercial success story which everyone seems to love to hate. Is it morally right to take advantage of patients' suffering? Should the drug companies exploit trivial symptoms by the widespread promotion of "cures" when the symptoms will subside anyway? Should doctors and their spouses be taken on lavish trips just because they are favourably disposed towards the drug company? Well, no, to all of these questions. These, though, are parodies of what really happens. Or are they?

Long life cycle of medicine

Most people know little about the life cycle of a medicine, but it is a complex story. Around one out of every 10,000 molecules tested or new concepts explored actually makes it to the clinical trial stage and then up to 14 years of research are needed before a substance receives a licence. Understandably, drug facts are easily forgotten so when, for example, the press decides to feature the impressive profits made by a successful pharmaceutical company, readers may all too easily believe that such a company is solely there to make massive amounts of money for its shareholders.

Let me therefore weigh the NHS's annual drug expenditure (£4.5 billion) against the annual net export of medicines from the UK (£4.9 billion), recognising, of course, that at the same time we import medicines and some raw materials. Let me also weigh the NHS's annual drug expenditure against its expenditure on everything else (more than £36 billion). Furthermore, without medicine some patients would require extra (costly) time in hospital or more expensive and maybe more risky procedures. Finally, let me weigh the £800 million profits made by pharmaceutical companies in the UK against the £400 million spent – allowed would be fairer – on promotion and, more importantly, against the £2 billion invested in research and development. So – commercial villain?

I hardly think so. Indeed, I am proud of having been part of a UK based success story, particularly given its positive contribution to the balance of trade and to Britain's economy.

Safety, efficacy and quality

Safety, efficacy, and quality are the factors on which the marketing authorisation of medicines is granted. Safety and efficacy, though, are relative, though interrelated factors. That means, for example, that for the very first treatment which is developed for a type of cancer which has hitherto been invariably rapidly fatal, the efficacy of the treatment might be quite low—though much better than nothing—while its safety profile might be horrendous. Such a product might rightly be allowed a licence because, on balance, for the patients for whom it is intended, it is likely to do significantly more good than harm. This is a commendable example of pragmatism working for the benefit of patients. By contrast, yet another new treatment for hypertension will not be granted a licence unless its safety potential is judged to be high.

Every medicine has to have a comprehensive safety database so that as much information as possible can be established about the safety of medicine in clinical practice. The industry is reasonably good at doing this, though companies are sometimes accused of mounting marketing exercises masquerading as clinical research, when what they are doing is undertaking essential studies, sometimes at the implied behest of the licensing authority. Companies certainly encourage better spontaneous reporting of adverse drug reactions by doctors to the Committee on Safety of Medicines than currently occurs. In fact, doctors are worse at reporting these than are the companies. If, however, the study is a marketing exercise in disguise then it is falling short of the promotional standards which apply across the industry and needs to be reported to the Prescription Medicines Code of Practice Authority. That only two cases have been found to have contravened the Code of Practice for the industry in this regard is encouraging.

Let me return to safety standards. The guidelines for the safety assessment of licensed medicines (SAMM), which were, to their credit, drafted by the industry in collaboration with the licensing authority and the medical profession, are nevertheless not ideal. They fail to recognise well enough the inevitable dilemma which arises when doctors are encouraged to report the experiences of their patients when prescribed a certain medicine, and are paid for doing so, against the need to establish an accurate safety profile for the medicine in question as quickly as possible. I acknowledge, though, that this will be a perceived conflict however good the guidelines become.

The industry has been actively involved in other people's standards where doing so has influenced its own. Thus, for example, it has been committed to supporting the training of research ethics committees, particularly because a greater understanding of the needs and expectations of both sides has been recognised as mutually valuable. It has also helped in the development of a training programme for clinical pharmacologists, providing for the first time within an approved programme a year's attachment to a pharmaceutical company. This participation acknowledges the value of industry expertise within this discipline as well as academic and NHS experience.

So my assessment of this half century of achievement by the pharmaceutical industry cannot be summarised as either just clinical saviour or commercial villain. To the NHS the industry has been a major contributor to the armamentarium of available treatment. To the country as a whole it has been a major commercial success. You cannot do much better than that.

A positive balance sheet

- The pharmaceutical industry of today, coping with mergers and takeovers, looks very different from the industry of 50 years ago: somewhat of a curate's egg, perhaps, but largely a fresh one, with the good overwhelmingly predominating.
- The net outcome from the industry during the 50 years of the NHS has been an impressive range of new treatments.
- The development of good standard treatments has not always been achieved without producing some dross, nor have the skills to use them ideally always been immediately or apparently available.
- The various voluntary and statutory controls have prevented financial exploitation, but the industry has been a financial as well as a medical success: overall, a positive balance sheet.

30:   General practice transformed

David Williams

In 1926, it was a home delivery. My father was not only present but "brought me into the world" himself. To buy house and practice in Wallasey, he had been fortunate in obtaining an interest free loan from a fellow Welshman. Father had served in the trenches with the Welsh Company of the Army Medical Corps. The older generation felt an enormous debt to those who survived.

He learned to apply forceps by practising at deliveries. There were few active drugs, no antibiotics, plenty of "TLC", little antenatal care, and no blood transfusion service. A blood stained note from a midwife would arrive at the dinner table. "She always manages to get blood on the note to emphasise the urgency," my father declared. Haemorrhage and infection were common and diphtheria antitoxin was kept in the car. Each district nurse was employed by a charity, a local district nursing association, and travelled by bicycle.

Patients who were not on the National Insurance "panel" had to pay. When the resident maids were not available, I would book in the money. Some patients were treated free. Lest they compared charges, entries in the daybook on the surgery desk were in a code, "Cumberland": ten letters, all different, to represent the figures from 0 to 9. The clerk to the local insurance committee moonlighted by sending out the monthly bills, and the new surgery suite, next door, attracted no government subsidy. Previously, patients had overflowed from the two waiting rooms onto the staircase. As a child, I had to climb over them.

Patients were accustomed to illness and death. Organic disease was respectable; the rest were "neurotics". Expectations were low and no one complained. At the Wallasey Cottage Hospital, GPs would operate on their own patients or give "rag and bottle" anaesthetics for the visiting surgical staff. These included Charles Wells (later Professor of Surgery at Liverpool) and C. McIntosh Marshall, whose book, in September 1939, promoted lower segment Caesarean section. GPs visited Highfield Maternity Hospital and the adjacent fever hospital – in that order. Because consultants were few and largely depended on GPs for their income, relations between them were close and contacts frequent.

Enter the NHS

There was no preregistration year for newly graduated doctors in 1949, so, before my first house post, I did GP locums in Wallasey. While I was acting for Dr Green, his partner, Dr Stewart-Hess, was called to a nursing home. He had to remove a placenta and asked me to administer chloroform (for the first time) but so profuse was the bleeding that the blood dripped down the patient's hair! With no obstetric flying squad, it was a great relief that we did not lose the mother. Neither of us forgot that day!

Financially, the NHS offered a regular income, some (deferred) "compensation" for the value of the GP's pre-NHS practice and no bad debts. So, in 1948, GPs cheerfully signed the deluge of application forms from patients, but most urban doctors lost their hospital connections and became more isolated from hospital medicine. The real gain lay in the removal of financial considerations from the consulting room. I am privileged to have practised medicine throughout the only period in medical history when patients could have complete confidence that treatment was offered solely on medical grounds. Before my day, patients had to consider the costs. After I retired, doctors had to do so. I had no private patients. I could give everyone, prince or pauper, the benefit of a therapeutic revolution so dramatic that the age structure of the population has been completely transformed.

Father decided to retire from Wallasey with his compensation to North Wales where, after a short interlude, he resumed work. So, in September 1954, after various hospital posts and two years as an RAF medical officer, I joined him in Holywell in partnership with Dr Gwilym Hooson. We were sometimes known, irreverently as "Father, Son and Holy Spirit". It was a real Trinity: three very different partners united in a common adventure. Neck glands were often tuberculous; Southey's tubes were used for cardiac failure; the malignant pustule of anthrax was diagnosed in the surgery; and a patient with open tuberculosis was found sleeping rough in the cattle market. We learned that medicine had a psychosocial dimension.

There was much to change. An interest free loan from the Group Practices Loan Fund helped us alter "Bodowen" and provide a new waiting room, a dispensary, and a flat for the caretaker. We introduced a child welfare clinic and, with the help of our farseeing Medical Officer of Health, Dr G. W. Roberts, pioneered the attachment of health visitors and district nurses to general practice in Flintshire. Through the Local Medical Committee, we demanded direct access to radiology and pathology services. Gwilym was a dynamic senior partner, much loved by his patients. Working with him and my father was a very special time.

Market town practice

Our rural dispensing practice covered 60 square miles. I would visit 20 or more patients each, but they would be in bed, upstairs, with soap, towel, and a bowl of hot water at the ready. There was no television to turn off but plenty of red flannel and goose grease to remove. In 1969, one elderly patient used an outside dry closet and relied on a land drain for her water. To the suggestion of a better house, she replied, "I'll get another bucket, Sir"!

Our practice premises, "Bodowen", had both history and character. The founder, Dr John Owen Jones, had lived and worked there. In 1895, Holywell had been labelled by one author Sewers End, because there was no drainage or fresh water system. A photograph in my possession shows a blind man with his donkey, selling water from a barrel outside "Bodowen"; another shows Dr Jones and his coachman in horse and trap.

Miss Edwards, the elderly and efficient dispenser, had been with the practice since qualifying. She had driven with Dr Jones in the trap and made up medicines by the fluid ounce in traditional corked bottles. No metrication for her. At night, she took the telephone calls and relayed them to the doctor. Patients did not argue with Miss Edwards. If one were to ask, "What's the medicine for?", he or she would be told, "It is to do you good!". Medical notes were brief and sometimes colourful. Hospital letters were filed in date order by hospital of origin. The practice included three branch surgeries, factory doctor work, beds in Holywell Cottage Hospital, and clinical assistantships in Lluesty General Hospital.

Lluesty had been a workhouse until 1948. Seven years later, the workhouse master had become hospital secretary and some of the former inmates were still housed in part III accommodation, treated by their own family doctors. The north wing was prison like, with wards radiating from a central point and, until a lift was installed, the narrow winding staircase made it difficult for ill patients to reach the wards or bodies to reach the mortuary. Gwilym questioned the fire precautions. There were three clinical assistants but no resident medical staff, so I usually worked from 9.00 am to 10.00 pm with breaks for meals. Outside those hours, "on call" duties were shared between Gwilym and myself. I remember a particularly horrific continuous period during the "Asian flu" outbreak when Gwilym, too, was ill for three weeks. The work was hard but offered great variety, plenty of interesting medicine and congenial patients.

Family Doctors' Charter

Dr George Eccleston succeeded my father in April 1962. He was a dedicated doctor and particularly interested in midwifery, establishing a joint clinic with the midwife and encouraging home deliveries. But GPs still needed tools, time, and training. Under the pool payment system, all expenses were refunded through gross pay. Doctors who spent least on their practices benefited most, and if Welsh doctors earned more from vaccination fees during an epidemic, all other GPs suffered a reduction of income! A letter to the *Sunday Times* in February 1965 suggested a pool system for Parliament:

> . . . the MPs' pool would be credited with (say) £3,000 per member together with the total expenses of all members as allowed by the Inland Revenue. There would be deducted from the pool any additional earnings received by members as ministers of the Crown or from trade union subsidies, city directorships, journalism and the like. The balance (if any) would be equally distributed between members. Those who became destitute could then console themselves with the knowledge that MPs as a group received a net annual average remuneration of £3,000 pa plus 100% refund of expenses. . .

The new charter for general practice in part solved the unfairness of the pool. After May 1966, direct reimbursement of rents, notional rents, rates, and up to 70% of the cost of ancillary staff, combined with a General Practice Finance Corporation (which lent money for premises) and, later, the cost-rent scheme, encouraged doctors to develop their practices and employ staff. In Holywell, we were able to introduce an appointment system, employ receptionists and house the attached district nurse-midwives and health visitor in the converted stable. The primary health care team had arrived and was underpinned by the introduction of vocational and postgraduate training

In January 1968, the Labour government reintroduced prescription charges. Because the Conservative Party was committed to exemptions for the old, the young, and the chronic sick, Labour could do no less. A joint working party between the Ministry of Health and the General Medical Services Committee (GMSC) which represented NHS GPs met to work out the details. Where does "acute" end and "chronic" begin? To ask GPs to draw such a fine line would reintroduce financial arguments into the consulting room.

As a member of the working party, I was unhappy with this, as were my colleagues. That is why we agreed an arbitrary and quite indefensible list of "chronic" conditions. The interim scheme was accepted by the profession on the Minister's strict assurance that a long term scheme involving plastic embossed cards would be put into effect as soon as possible. The interim scheme still operates in 1997.

Welsh input

Welsh doctors contributed to the renaissance of general practice through the Welsh Royal College of General Practitioners and General Medical Services Committee (WGMSC). Research papers were published, among which Dr Julian Tudor Hart's contribution was outstanding. In 1972,

WGMSC presented "Long term policies in general practice" to the GPs' annual conference. The conference adopted the strategy, which included moves to bring family planning, child health and computing fully within general practice. The Welsh committee also launched medical audit into general practice in 1976, when our joint report with our consultant colleagues, "Medical audit by peer review", was sent to all local medical committees. Unfortunately, it did not mature quite as we had planned – but that is democracy for you.

The development of community hospitals was close to our hearts. Doctors in Mold and Deeside even managed to acquire new ones, but Holywell still waits! Even so, led by Dr Arthur Roberts, the practice has built a magnificent new "Bodowen", which I h the great pleasure of opening in 1993.

Compassion losing out to bureaucracy

As the NHS celebrates its 50th birthday, rationing of health care is high on its agenda.

- Who is to be held accountable for deciding that correcting this patient's infertility is essential but replacing that patient's hip is not? No one wants the job: it is a poisoned chalice.
- In 1948, the Second World War had accustomed everyone to value duty to the community above the selfish exercise of individual "rights" and wishes, but by 1997 the consumer society had reversed that ethos, causing patients to demand medical care like instant coffee.
- The old restraints have gone, so demand is increasingly contained by inflexible rules and rigid cash limits; decisions become anonymous and capricious and local, not national.
- Mutual trust and appreciation are reduced and there is less room for compassion, that bedrock of medicine. Bureaucracy rules.
- To preserve our NHS and our planet, we must abandon consumerism and retrieve our sense of community.
- If rationing of health care is necessary, let it be based on community values and the views of the whole community.

Selected chronology of twentieth century events in the development and provisions of comprehensive health care in the United Kingdom*

For an institution as large, complex and constantly changing as the UK's National Health Service, preparing a chronology was inevitably a highly selective process. The responsibility for the events chosen and their accuracy is mine. I drew on many sources but would like to acknowledge in particular Peter Bartrip's *Themselves Writ Large: The BMA 1832-1996*; Rudolf Klein's *The New Politics of the NHS*; Geoffrey Rivett's *From Cradle to Grave: 50 years of the NHS*; Nicholas Timmins's *The Five Giants: a biography of the Welfare State*; Charles Webster's *The Health Services Since the War*, *The British Medical Journal* and *The History of the British Medical Association, Vol II*; *The NHS - A Kaleidoscope of Care - Conflicts of Service and Business Values*, of which I was co-author with Tony Kember.

Gordon Macpherson
Editor

The first half century

1907   School Medical Service set up.

1911   National Insurance Act passed in the wake of a Royal Commission's proposal: basic structure of general practitioner and pharmaceutical services laid down for working population.

---

* Health care in Scotland and Northern Ireland developed broadly in parallel with that in England and Wales, though legislation was customarily separately enacted to take account of national requirements.

1913   Ministry of Health set up.

1920   Report from the government's Council of Medical and Allied Services (chaired by the physician Lord Dawson of Penn) recommended plans to develop a comprehensive and unified health service based on health centres.

1926   Royal Commission on National Health Insurance suggested government funding of health services.

1929   Poor Law scheme ended and responsibility for health care for poor shifted to local government, which became prime provider of hospital and (some) community care.

1930   Mental Treatment Act passed, a reforming legislative landmark in mental health care.
The British Medical Association (BMA) published a plan for general medical services funded by an extension of the National Insurance scheme.

1933   The BMA published a report on nutrition that recommended specimen diets: diet, nutrition and health brought to forefront of public consciousness.

1936   In response to official concerns about the population's health and physical fitness, a BMA inquiry called for measures to improve nation's health through better physical recreation; physical fitness deserved recognition alongside housing, sanitation and nutrition as one of "great social services" vital to public health.

1937   Government legislation followed the BMA's report on physical fitness.

1938   The BMA published a revised version of its 1930 report on *General Medical Service for the Nation.*

1939   Emergency Medical Service set up to integrate Britain's hospital services to cope with wartime demands.

On 3 September Britain declared war against Germany.

1942   On 1 December the Coalition Government published a report *Social Insurance and Allied Services* prepared by the econmist, academic and civil servant William Beveridge. The Beveridge report, aimed at combatting the "five giants" of "Want, Disease, Ignorance, Squalor and Idleness", became the template for the post war, "cradle to grave" Welfare State and included proposals for a national health service.

1944   The Coalition Government published a White Paper on a national health service and entered discussions with interested parties including the medical profession.

1945   Second World War ended. Labour Government elected with large majority in July; Aneurin Bevan appointed Minister of Health and Housing.

1946   New government introduced National Health Service Bill, which received Royal Assent in November. Tripartite service proposed comprising a hospital service, family practitioner services and local government based public health and schools medical services.

1947   Medical profession opposed aspects of the NHS Act and BMA entered negotiations with Aneurin Bevan. Presidents of Royal Colleges discussed proposed NHS with the Minister.

1948   Negotiations between BMA and government deadlocked; February plebiscite of all doctors showed 75% of profession opposed to working in NHS as planned by the government.

Aneurin Bevan promised to amend the 1946 NHS Act to take account of doctors' concerns about clinical independence, remuneration structure and private practice.

In May the BMA recommended doctors to cooperate with the new service.

5 July: NHS inaugurated, patients flocked to use its services.

1949   First signs of funding difficulties as patients' demands on the service greatly exceeded estimates, thus pushing costs to worrying levels.

Pre 1948 GPs' interests had been represented by Insurance Acts Committee of BMA; this was replaced by General Medical Services Committee, an autonomous committee of the BMA. The association set up a consultants' committee to represent their medicopolitical interests. The Royal Colleges remained a powerful source of expert advice.

The 1950s

1950   Labour Government re-elected with majority of six. Rising costs of NHS continued to alarm the Treasury, spending limit imposed.

Report on general practice by New Zealand trained general practitioner Joseph Collings, commissioned in 1948 by Nuffield Provincial Hospitals Trust, highlighted great variations in quality among 55 English practices; it stimulated wide debate and a clutch of other reports.

Committee chaired by physician Sir Henry Cohen set up to examine general practice. Reporting in 1954, it concluded that general practice was a special branch of medicine for which practitioners should have three years of supervised training.

1951   In January Bevan moved to Ministry of Labour and in April resigned from the Cabinet over imposition of charges for dental treatment and spectacles: the completely free and comprehensive health service had ended.

New Minister of Health, Hilary Marquand, no longer in Cabinet, and with Bevan's departure the ministry's power in Whitehall waned.

October General Election resulted in a Conservative Government; it supported the NHS's principles but was concerned about how to fund rising demands, particularly for medicines. Harry Crookshank appointed Minister of Health.

1952   A government initiated review of general practitioners' pay, undertaken by Lord Justice Dankwerts, proposed massive increase: £40 million in back pay (10% of total annual cost of NHS) and £10 million a year extra for GPs. The Cabinet reluctantly accepted this.

Ian Macleod appointed Minister of Health.

College of General Practitioners founded despite reservations of some of Royal Colleges.

A 1s 0d (5p) prescription charge introduced.

1953   Government set up inquiry, chaired by economist Claude Guillebaud, to inquire into rising cost of NHS.

1954   The BMA asked the government for an inquiry into medical manpower because it feared a surplus of doctors.

Bradbeer Committee on hospital administration recommended hospital medical staff committees and a single administrative officer (not a doctor) at group (hospital management committee) level.

1955   Conservative Government returned to power at election. Robert Turton appointed Minister of Health.

1956   Guillebaud report defended the structure and costs of NHS, pointing out that as a proportion of gross domestic product cost of services had been falling.

Clean Air Act passed.

1957   Recurrent disputes between successive governments and doctors over latters' pay led to appointment of Royal Commission to review doctors' and dentists' pay, chaired by industrialist Sir Harry Pilkington.

Dennis Vosper appointed Minister of Health in January and replaced by Derek Walker-Smith in September.

Royal Commission on mental illness reported calling for a single new law to cover all mental disorders, the removal of distinctions between physical and mental illness and the treatment of those with mental illness to be carried out in the community where possible.

Willink report on medical manpower, published by the government, recommended 10% cut in number of graduates.

1958   BMA initiated a professional based inquiry, chaired by surgeon Sir Arthur Porritt, to review "whole field of publicly administered medical services".

Former Tory minister of health Ian McLeod claimed that "The National Health Service, with the exception of recurring spasms about charges, is out of party politics."

Introduction of 44 hour working week for nurses.

1959　New Mental Health Act launched the reorientation of the mental health services from institutional to community based care.

Conservative Government reelected with majority of 100.

Hinchcliffe and Douglas (Scotland) Committees reviewed rising prescribing costs: both opposed limited list of NHS drugs, and former opposed prescription charges.

Maternity Services Committee (an official body) recommended greater cooperation and coordination within the maternity services, with a hospital delivery rate of 70% suggested.

1960s

1960　Royal Commission on Doctors' and Dentists' Remuneration reported: it recommended establishment of an independent pay review system for the two professions as well as a substantial pay rise. Government and BMA accepted report.

1961　Government initiated report on medical staffing structure in the hospital service, chaired by Sir Robert Platt, recommended an increase in consultant establishment and introduction of subconsultant grade (medical assistants).

1962　Porritt report recommended integration of tripartite structure of NHS, with area boards set up to run the service.

Enoch Powell published *Hospital Plan for England and Wales*, a planned capital investment programme of £500 million to launch a network of district general hospitals; the 10 year plan aimed to replace 750 of existing 2,000 hospitals in England and Wales. Scotland had a similar plan.

Royal College of Physicians published landmark report linking smoking and ill health.

Committee on Safety of Drugs set up to devise a system of assessing new drugs in the wake of the disaster with the sleeping drug thalidomide; introduced in 1956 this was found to cause congenital deformities in babies whose mothers had taken it during pregnancy.

1963　First report of professions' pay review body recommended increase of 14%; GPs dissatisfied because "pool" system of remuneration produced unfair distribution of expenses.

Gillie report on general practice emphasised importance of post-graduate education and endorsed group practice.

Anthony Barber appointed Minister of Health. He set up joint ministerial/professional working party on general practice (Fraser).

1964   Salmon Committee on senior nurse staffing structure recommended new hospital grading system based on first line, middle and top management; proposals implemented in 1966.

Labour Government elected with small majority in October 1964. Kenneth Robinson appointed Minister of Health.

1965   Dissatisfaction among general practitioners about pay structure led to threats of resignation from NHS. Negotiations started with Kenneth Robinson based on proposals in profession's *Charter for the Family Doctor Service*.

Royal Commission on medical education set up.

Government abolished prescription charges.

December 1965, government set up Seebohm Committee to review personal social services.

1966   Labour Government reelected with bigger majority: Kenneth Robinson remained Minister of Health.

Government and BMA agreed a new contract for general practitioners: greater investment in primary care and much improved pay led to sustained renaissance in general practice.

1967   BMA sent memorandum to government on problems of hospital medical staff - described as "Hospital Doctors' Charter".

Rising concern about supply of doctors, in particular emigration of UK trained doctors and NHS's increasing dependence on doctors from abroad, mainly the Indian subcontinent.

"Cogweel" report on organisation of medical work in hospitals. Prepared by a joint ministerial/professional working party, it

187

proposed a structure of clinical divisions headed by a small representative medical executive committee.

David Steel's private member's Bill to legalise abortion (subject to certain criteria) approved by Parliament.

Sans everything, a report on behalf of a charity for the elderly, was a devastating critique of conditions in long stay institutions; along with subsequent critical reports this eventually prodded the government into action (see 1969).

Health Education Council established.

1968   Ministry of Health merged with Ministry of Social Security under new Secretary of State (Richard Crossman) with seat in Cabinet.

Government Green Papers on changes in administrative structure of NHS proposed unification of hospital and community health services under area health boards.

Seebohm Committee recommended radical shake up of social service training and organisation: profound implications for medical care.

Royal Commission on Medical Education (Todd report) recommended a rise in numbers of medical schools and students, increasing annual intake to 3,700 by 1975, an interim target on the way to a preferred figure of 5,000 by 1985-9. Government backed 3,700 target.

Hospital doctors and Department of Health and Social Security (DHSS) completed negotiations on charter.

Medicines Act 1968 passed in October consolidated and extended legislation on the safety, quality and efficacy of medicinal products as well as regulation of sales and promotion. It set up the Medicines Commission and a licensing system.

Prescription charges reintroduced.

1969   Richard Crossman warns of the "truly terrifying" prospects of the rising costs of the Welfare State: DHSS appointed its first two economists, mainly because of anxieties about the effect of technology on NHS costs.

Extra duty allowances introduced for hospital junior staff in recognition of long hours of work.

In June Royal Commission on Local Government proposed 58 unitary local authorities, suggesting also that local government assumed responsibility for NHS. Neither proposal accepted.

Green Paper on reorganisation of health and social services in Northern Ireland.

Bonham-Carter report on functions of district general hospitals.

Public disquiet about conditions in Ely Hospital Cardiff, a long stay institution for mentally ill and handicapped patients, prompted an official inquiry led by Geoffrey Howe QC. A devastating indictment of the hospital was the forerunner of a decade of scandals about the state of NHS long stay hospitals. The Howe report led to immediate establishment of the independent Hospital Advisory Service (Scotland had its own), which sent inspectorial/advisory teams to long stay hospitals and published reports on the findings.

The 1970s

1970   Second Green Paper on NHS reorganisation published.

Labour Government refused to implement in full Review Body's pay award to doctors and dentists. BMA imposed sanctions; Review Body resigned.

Local Authority Social Services Act 1970 became law: local authorities required to create unified social service departments in April 1971; new training arrangements planned.

Conservative Government elected in June. Sir Keith Joseph succeeded Richard Crossman as Secretary of State for NHSS.

New government re-established independent Review Body and implemented previous pay recommendations.

In November nurses asked for a pay rise and cut in working hours that represented an increase of 27%; this was in addition to a 20% rise introduced in April.

1971   Consultative Document on NHS reorganisation in England published.

BMA registered as a trade union (special register) under government's industrial relations legislation.

White Papers on improving services for mentally ill and handicapped people proposed inpatient units in district hospitals along with expanded community care.

1972   Sir Keith Joseph published White Paper on NHS reorganisation proposing unification of hospital and community health services.

Nearly 100,000 ancillary staff in NHS went on strike for higher pay, the first extensive industrial action in the service.

Briggs report on nursing proposed lowered entry age, restructure of training and improved career structure.

Government launched inquiry into General Medical Council following public and professional dissatisfaction with its workings.

1973   NHS Reorganisation Act passed introducing area and district boards which were to run hospital and community health services by consensus management as laid down in the 'Grey Book', *Management Arrangements for the reorganised NHS*, a document agreed between the Department of Health and staff representatives. Public given a voice through community health councils. Health Service Commissioner (Ombudsman) appointed.

United Kingdom joined European Common Market and BMA became full member of Standing Committee of Doctors.

Unrest over pay among nurses and ancillary workers led to the latter targeting major hospitals with selective strike action: unions eventually settled for modest government concessions. Nurses' dissatisfaction persisted, aggravated by delay in implementing the 1972 Briggs report.

1974   Conservative Government's pay policy caused discontent not only among NHS staff but among a wide range of workers including the miners. Confrontation with the miners led to General Election in February and fall of the government. Labour Party took office, but with a minority in Parliament. Further election in October gave Labour Party a majority of three.

Barbara Castle appointed Secretary of State for Social Services.

On 1 April NHS's administrative structure reorganised into three tiers: local authority involvement restricted to environmental services, with other public health responsibilities transferred to NHS. In England 14 regional health authorities, 90 area health authorities and 200 district management teams replaced old tripartite structure. Hospital and community health services run by consensus management; family practitioner services remained separate.

Local government reorganised: 400 local authorities replaced 1,700, but attempts to achieve coterminosity with new health authorities failed.

Government set up inquiry into pay and conditions of service of nurses and professions supplementary to medicine chaired by Lord Halsbury.

In July BMA, British Dental Association and Royal Colleges of Nurses and of Midwives warned the government of imminent collapse of NHS because of cuts in funding. Professions' leaders met Prime Minister to ask for more resources and an independent inquiry into funding. He refused.

Consultants took industrial action in defence of pay beds in NHS, which new government planned to abolish, a policy strongly backed by health service unions.

1975 Pay beds dispute remained deadlocked: Prime Minister Harold Wilson eventually asked Lord Goodman to mediate. Compromise achieved (in early 1976) but only after consultants had renewed sanctions. These coincided with sanctions imposed by hospital junior staff, who had fallen out with the government over new "closed end" contracts which the BMA had negotiated but which "grass roots" junior doctors criticised as unsatisfactory.

In July Barbara Castle met a delegation from the health professions,

191

who remained perturbed about state of NHS. In October, with the junior doctors' problems still unresolved, the Prime Minister promised a Royal Commission on the NHS. Chaired by Sir Alec Merrison, this started work in 1976.

Formula devised by Department of Health's Resource Allocation Working Party (RAWP) to redistribute NHS resources from "over endowed" regions - the four Thames RHAs - to poorer parts of NHS. Planning system for NHS proposed.

Merrison committee reviewing workings of General Medical Council reported with wide ranging proposals for reform in the regulation of the medical profession.

1976   Dispute between the government and junior doctors over hours of work and extra duty payments rumbled on until September when agreement was reached and industrial action stopped.

Goodman proposals on private practice in NHS approved by consultants, who suspended sanctions; subsequent *Health Services Act 1976* enacted the proposals, which under supervision of independent board cut private NHS beds in NHS hospitals. Negotiations resumed on a new work sensitive consultant contract.

Court report on future of child health services published.

Hospital Advisory Service was transmuted into Health Advisory Service with a consequential broader remit.

In April Barbara Castle was succeeded by David Ennals as Secretary of State for Social Services.

Department of Health published planning paper *Priorities for Health and Personal Social Services in England*, which warned that economic limitations meant choices in health care had to be made. Cash limits extended to most NHS spending.

Serious crisis in Britain's economy led to severe cuts in public expenditure as a condition for obtaining loan from International Monetary Fund. NHS spending plans pruned.

The White Paper, *Prevention and Health*, published in December, signalled the government's greater commitment to the prevention of ill health; even so, funding of Health Education Council remained inadequate.

1977   Mounting adverse publicity over closure of NHS facilities spurred Secretary of State Ennals to campaign within Whitehall for immediate injection of £30 million and for a target growth rate of 3% annual increase in NHS budget. Small improvements achieved for 1977-9 budgets.

Government published *The Way Forward*, the outcome of its 1976 consultative document on priorities.

London Health Planning Consortium set up to rationalise the capital's complex health services.

Concern that deprived regions were not getting their share of resources prompted Ennals to set up working group, chaired by Sir Douglas Black, Chief Scientist at the Department of Health, to investigate inequalities in health.

A report on community health councils concluded that despite failures, frustration and "puny resources", the councils continued to thrive and were capable of "even more ambitious functions".

1978   Medical Act 1978 reconstituted General Medical Council and gave the council new powers to control registration of doctors unfit to practise.

5 July: Government issued "celebratory" booklet on thirty years of the NHS. Meanwhile waiting lists were rising to record levels.

Government published discussion paper, *Medical Manpower - The Next Twenty Years*.

The government's incomes policy came under increasing pressure with industrial militancy among the public sector workers, including NHS staff, rising. The Doctors' and Dentists' Review Body proposed substantial increases plus a two stage catching up award of 18%. In the autumn other health workers demanded large pay rises despite a 10% award earlier in the year.

1979   As 1978 gave way to 1979 anger among public sector workers, including NHS staff, worsened, and the period was dubbed the "winter of discontent" with unemployment reaching politically damaging levels and industrial action in NHS continuing. Nine percent pay rises for non-medical NHS staff and promise of a pay inquiry (Clegg) cooled staff unrest. Despite cuts in government spending, the NHS escaped largely unscathed. With the effects of RAWP beginning to bite, however, the consequences for health services continued the air of crisis that had been a feature since 1976.

The BMA's General Medical Services Committee published a new charter for general practice calling for more doctors and more investment for primary care, better vocational training, medical audit, extension of GPs' services and a more work sensitive contract with greater rewards.

James Callaghan's minority Labour Government went to the polls in May and was defeated. Margaret Thatcher became Prime Minster in the Tory Government.

In July 1979 the Royal Commission on the NHS reported, overwhelmingly endorsing the NHS. It criticised, however, the excess of administrative tiers and administrators and warned that money was being wasted. Among its 117 recommendations, it urged a strengthening of regional health authorities, the abolition of family practitioner committees and the inclusion of general practice in the mainstream of the NHS. The new government's response was low key.

Consultants rejected the Review Body's pricing of the contract agreed between the BMA and Labour's David Ennals. A revised contract was negotiated with Patrick Jenkin, the new Secretary of State: this allowed full time consultants to do some private practice and modified existing part time contracts. The Government also abolished the Health Services Board and encouraged new pay beds in NHS hospitals.

In December the Department of Health issued a consultative document on NHS reorganisation, *Patients First*. It proposed simplification of the NHS structure: area health authorities were to be replaced by district authorities as the central tier; regional health authorities survived but the Royal Commission's proposal to strengthen them was not incorporated. The government wanted decisions taken as near to the point of delivery as possible. Consensus management 1974 style was downplayed and the input of professional and other special interest groups reduced.

The 1980s

1980   The Health Services Act 1980 translated into legislation the proposals for reorganising the NHS contained in the 1979 consultative document (see above). The changes would be introduced in 1982.

A Department of Health document on the future of NHS hospital services rejected the concept of large district general hospitals, decreeing a maximum size of 600 beds, while praising the value of small hospitals.

The number of people covered by private health insurance rose by 26%, a rate of increase that fell to 13% in 1981. The Minister of Health, Dr Gerard Vaughan, forecast that 20% of the population would have private cover by 1985, a comment that tempted several American health organisations to enter the British health care market.

The Black report *Inequalities in Health*, commissioned by Ennals in 1977 (see above), was published. It showed that death rates from many illnesses were higher for the lower social and occupational classes than for social classes I and II. Despite the Welfare State and the NHS the health gap between the poor and the better off was widening. The authors proposed better benefits and an emphasis on prevention of ill health. The potential costs prompted Patrick Jenkin to reject the report, but it was to remain an influential social document.

1981   In September Norman Fowler succeeded Patrick Jenkin as Secretary of State. He halted a departmental inquiry into alternative health service finance, arguing that whatever system was used taxation would still have to fund most health care.

The government published *Care in Action*, its priorities for the NHS: like its predecessors the document earmarked services for the elderly, mentally handicapped and other deprived groups as a priority. The government advocated cooperation between public and private sectors and emphasised its aim of simplifying and decentralising services.

The BMA backed medical audit organised and administered by doctors.

Publication of report on primary care in London prepared by Professor Donald Acheson (later to be appointed Chief Medical Officer).

1982   Non-medical NHS staff had in 1981 reluctantly accepted a 6% pay rise and a cut in the nurses' working week. For 1982 the Royal College of Nursing and the TUC-linked health unions demanded 12% rises. The unions organised one day strikes to back their demands while the RCN ran a high profile publicity campaign. This proved a powerful political challenge to the government. By offering marginal improvements and, importantly, an independent pay review body for nurses, midwives and other health professionals, ministers eventually persuaded staff to end their eight months of disruption, which had resulted in a 100,000 rise in hospital waiting lists to 720,000.

In April the NHS underwent its second major reorganisation with the cumbersome 1974 structure being slimmed down by the abolition of area health authorities. The changes broadly followed the proposals in the 1979 consultative document (see above).

As part of its policy to contain rising NHS costs the Department of Health asked Binder Hamlyn, a firm of financial accountants, to study the feasibility of applying cash limits to family practitioner services. Since 1948 the budget for these services had been largely demand led. Though the report was never published it was understood to have proposed larger capitation fees and a cut in item of service payments, and the findings informed subsequent policy decisions.

1982 saw the expiry of the Tory Government's pledge to honour its predecessor's three year NHS spending plans from 1979. This, combined with the introduction of cash instead of volume planning and demands on health authorities to generate annual savings of up to 1% of their cash limits, meant much tighter financial discipline in the NHS. Annual performance reviews of all tiers of the service coupled with performance indicators were also introduced.

Norman Fowler again stated that taxation would remain the predominant way of financing the NHS, and the Prime Minister told the Tory's annual conference: "Let me make one thing absolutely clear. The National Health Service is safe with us".

The BMA and the government started discussions to limit the cost of medicines by the use of generic instead of branded drugs.

The first of six reports from the official Körner inquiry into health services information appeared. These reports would influence the development of information technology.

Compulsory vocational training introduced for intending general practitioners.

Conservative Government elected for its second term of office.

1983   The government initiated a review of the management of the NHS. Roy Griffiths, managing director of a supermarket, and three other experienced businessmen spent six months roaming the NHS. Then they produced a brief report that was to revolutionise the management of the health service. They called for the establishment of the general management function with better management training, particularly for doctors and nurses. General managers would be held accountable for their performance. The politics and policies of the NHS would be the Department of Health's responsibility while a new management arm of the department would manage the service and implement the policies. Despite reservations among staff, the government readily accepted the Griffiths proposals and implemented them over the succeeding two years.

The Department of Health instituted competitive tendering, with all health authorities required to test the cost effectiveness of all cleaning, catering and laundering services.

United Kingdom Central Council for Nursing, Midwifery and Health Visiting (UKCC) set up following legislation in 1979 that reflected recommendations of the 1972 Briggs report on nursing.

The BMA's general practitioner committee published *General Practice: a British success* which promised to support improved co-ordination and integration in the NHS and called for an expansion of general practice.

In December Kenneth Clarke, Minister for Health, announced restrictions on the use of deputising services by general practitioners, a step taken without the prior consultation with the profession that customarily preceded such announcements. The BMA reacted angrily but, with some alterations, the new rules were introduced in

197

1984.

Nurses' independent pay review body started work.

Health Care and Its Costs, a government document published just before the General Election, showed that productivity had risen faster than resources between 1976 and 1981.

1984 The Griffiths management reforms began to be implemented (see 1983).

The pressure for efficiency savings from the Conservative Government had resulted in around £50 million saved between 1981 and 1983. In 1984 the Department of Health introduced a more stringent cost improvement programme (CIP), which achieved greater savings.

Health ministers initiated a departmental review of the family practitioner services.

The Health and Social Security Act 1984 tightened up the responsibilities of health and local authorities for regulating the private sector, which was increasingly providing institutional care for the steadily increasing number of elderly people. This social, health and financial issue was to become a major concern of governments and the public.

Government set up Warnock inquiry to examine issues surrounding techniques for modifying human reproductive processes.

Health Minister Clarke announced a limited list of drugs - excluding brand name medicines considered too expensive or too ineffective to be provided by the NHS. No prior consultation with the BMA had taken place. The result was major conflict between GPs and the Department of Health. After modification a compromise scheme was introduced in 1985 and proved generally successful. The episode was a watershed in relations between the profession and a government which thereafter increasingly downgraded the input of professional advice in the formation of government policies on the NHS.

1985 The limited list of NHS prescribable drugs was introduced.

The Royal College of General Practitioners published its strategy for raising quality in primary care - *Towards quality in general practice* - and analysed the character of good practice in *What sort of doctor?*.

A monograph commissioned by the Nuffield Provincial Hospital Trust, *Reflections on the Management of the NHS,* was published. Written by Professor Alain Enthoven, an American health expert, it attracted limited attention but was to prove influential in shaping the Conservative Government's subsequent internal market reforms of the NHS.

The Institute of Health Services Management, the RCN and the BMA collaborated in commissioning a report on the financial prospects for the NHS. They called for annual 2% growth, more flexibility for health authorities to plan their budgets and warned that the NHS was seriously underfunded.

Family practitioner committees were given independent status.

Cumberledge inquiry into community nursing launched.

1986   On 21 April the Conservative Government issued its first big initiative on primary care. *Primary Health Care: an agenda for discussion* set six objectives: more consumer responsive services; higher standards of care; promotion of health and prevention of illness; greater choice for patients; better value for money; and clearer priorities for the family practitioner services. To help achieve these aims the government proposed controversial changes in the structure of GPs' remuneration including a "good practice allowance" and raising the proportion paid by capitation fees while reducing that paid through item of service fees. It rejected cash limits but looked for ways to limit expenditure.

The discussion document proposed changes to dentists' contracts with the introduction of capitation fees. Reform was also planned for pharmacists' NHS work, which had already been under review. The government also suggested that pharmacists should extend their role, including advising patients on minor symptoms.

The Cumberledge report on community nursing, published simultaneously with the primary care Green Paper, called for resources to be switched from hospitals to the community, the development of nurse practitioners, better training for community nurses and the freedom for nurses to do some prescribing.

For the sixth consecutive year the government interfered with the recommendations of the independent review body on doctors' and dentists' pay, once again prompting questions in the professions about its value.

Since 1948 nursing had undergone radical changes with nurses becoming more autonomous, adopting the nursing process and undertaking many technical activities. The UKCC wanted to raise the quality of nursing and launched Project 2000 to achieve this by moving from the traditional apprentice type training to an American style academic course. It was to be introduced amidst some controversy in 1988.

The Audit Commission published an incisive analysis of community care, *Making a reality of community care*, that highlighted the gaps developing in the mental health services because the run down in hospital beds was not being matched by the necessary expansion of community services. Local authorities provided a "very uneven pattern" of service. Reporting that the reduction in NHS beds for the elderly had been offset by the growth in private residential homes, the commission warned that the cost to the Exchequer (via welfare benefits) was £500 million in 1986 (a figure that would rise to over £2 billion over the next 10 years or so). Much of the £6 billion a year for services for the mentally ill and handicapped and the elderly was being misspent, according to the commission.

In December, when the Audit Commission's report appeared, the Prime Minister invited Sir Roy Griffiths - now her special adviser on health - "to find a solution to the problems of community care".

The Department of Health launched the resource management initiative to introduce clinical budgeting into hospitals, at first in six pilots. Resource management aimed to link cost effective performance, information provision and managerial participation and process. It led to the establishment of clinical directorates, an American system pioneered in 1985 in Britain at Guy's Hospital, London.

1987 Publication of a joint Health Department/medical profession report, *Hospital Medical Staffing: Achieving a Balance*. The culmination of years of arguments about how to match training posts to career opportunities in the specialities while reducing junior doctors' long hours of work, the report suggested measures to promote expansion of consultant establishment, to control the number of training posts and to introduce a new career post of staff grade. Despite a controversial reception the reforms were introduced, only to be complicated by the Conservative Government's subsequent introduction of the internal market in 1991 and the 1993 Calman report on specialist training.

A White Paper, *Promoting Better Health*, while modifying some of the proposals in the 1986 Green Paper on primary care, was broadly consistent with most of its ideas; it was the start of tough negotiations on the future of primary care.

A survey showing an extremely high level of dissatisfaction among nurses prompted the government to earmark £800 million for a clinical regrading exercise. Underestimates of the cost, an unrealistic timetable, the lack of consultation with health authorities and a shortage of competent assessors led to delays, with managers frustrated and nurses angry. Eventually implemented, the Government claimed in 1992 that it had doubled the time that NHS trained nurses stayed in the service.

Conservative Government reelected in June with reduced majority.

John Moore succeeded Norman Fowler - the longest serving health minister in the NHS - as Secretary of State for Social Services. He was faced with a worsening financial crisis, the result of five years of funding restraints, including enforced efficiency savings and despite CIP (see 1984) and competitive tendering (see 1983). Health authorities were surviving by closing beds and deferring the payment of bills. The NHS was said to be technically bankrupt.

The BMA, the Institute of Health Service Management and the RCN again commissioned an independent academic review into the NHS's financial position. The outcome was a recommendation to link NHS funding to growth in national income with provisions made for demographic changes and treatment of major new diseases (for example, AIDS). The three organisations estimated that over three years an extra £1.7 billion would be required.

Regional general managers and chairmen joined the warning chorus about a financial crisis and, unusually, presidents of the three senior Royal Colleges personally met the Prime Minister to emphasise the gravity of the crisis.

1988   In January the Prime Minister announced during a television interview that a review of the NHS was underway, news that

201

surprised ministers and civil servants. The review was led by her and membership included five ministers and Sir Roy Griffiths.

Sir Roy Griffiths' commissioned review of community care, *Community Care: Agenda for Action*, was delivered to the government at the start of the year but because its recommendations were unpalatable to the Prime Minister, publication was deferred until just after Chancellor Lawson's much publicised 1988 budget. It was treated as a consultation document: Griffiths proposed that local authorities should act as purchasing agents for community care services many of which should be provided in people's own homes. The government promised to publish its own proposals later.

The Prime Minister's high level review of the NHS continued almost in secret, with no formal outside evidence called for and amidst rumours of sharp divisions among ministers. John Moore was unwell and Kenneth Clarke replaced him as Secretary of State for Health in June, when social security responsibilities were hived off as a separate department.

The government published *Public Health in England*: this emphasised the need for adequate health care assessment, the AIDS epidemic having alerted the public and politicians to the value of "public health", an essential part of a comprehensive health service and one which had suffered years of neglect.

Start of national breast screening programme of women. Recommended in the government commissioned Forrest report of 1986, it covered the age groups 50 to 64 years.

1989   On 31 January the Government published *Working for Patients*, the White Paper containing proposals for reforming the NHS produced by the Prime Minister's review team. Kenneth Clarke publicly launched the document at a large meeting of NHS managers and other professionals, his aim being to cascade information on the proposed changes down through the NHS as quickly as possible. The White Paper announced the introduction of an internal market for the NHS, with purchasers (health authorities and general practitioners) contracting with providers (hospital and community health services operating as locally based independent trusts) to provide services required by patients in the purchasers' areas of responsibility. A radical innovation was to enable general practitioners who wished to do so to become fundholders: they would be given budgets to purchase secondary non-acute services. Government wanted the changes to be implemented in April 1991, an ambitious timetable for such fundamental changes.

The White Paper provoked strong opposition, in particular from the Labour Party and the BMA, both of which feared that the internal market would destroy the comprehensive, integrated character of the NHS. They doubted the government's assurance that the service would remain primarily tax financed and that privatisation was not the ultimate objective. The BMA launched a high profile publicity campaign against the White Paper: though it had an impact on the public, the campaign failed to stop the government's plans.

1989 saw the continuation of discussions between the government and the BMA over a new contract for general practitioners based on the consumer oriented proposals in the 1986 White Paper. Since the profession preferred the status quo, discussions were prolonged and difficult. After the GPs' leaders and Kenneth Clarke finally struck a deal in May at a 10 hour meeting, GPs overwhelmingly rejected it in a countrywide ballot. The Secretary of State nevertheless implemented the contract. The negotiations and implementation of the contract were complicated by the plans for fundholding general practices in *Working for Patients*.

Caring for People: community care in the next decade and beyond, a White Paper published in July, was the government's response to the Griffiths' proposals on community care (1988), which, because the author wanted local authorities to act as agents for purchasing care, had not been welcomed by the Cabinet. Nevertheless, *Caring for People* accepted that local authorities' social services departments should be the lead agencies. Its recommendations were to be incorporated in the legislation to reform the NHS.

The Department of Health launched the income generation initiative aimed at persuading hospitals to make better commercial use of their assets - for example, by renting out space for shops and fully utilising their facilities for private patients.

The General Practice Finance Corporation - the successful initiative from the 1966 charter negotiations which enabled GPs to borrow money for buying or improving premises - was converted into a limited company, thus removing it from the public expenditure sector.

The 1990s

1990   The National Health Service and Community Care Act 1990 was passed: few changes were introduced during its passage through Parliament, and the internal market was set to start on 1 April 1991.

The new contract for general practitioners was introduced; many GPs were still opposed to it but, unlike 1965, they did not support collective action to resist the changes. The General Medical Services Committee, which represents all NHS GPs, decided instead to monitor the working of the contract.

Margaret Thatcher, worried about the widespread opposition to her NHS reforms and politically unsettled by the Trafalgar Square riots accompanying the introduction of the community charge (poll tax) in the Spring, asked a small group of businessmen to tour the NHS and assess whether the NHS reforms would work. Despite their doubts Kenneth Clarke adamantly refused to postpone the changes, but the changes to community care arrangements incorporated in the 1990 Act were deferred until 1993 because of practical and financial problems.

Margaret Thatcher was displaced as Prime Minister by John Major. William Waldegrave replaced Kenneth Clarke as Secretary of State for Health.

The first director of research and development in the NHS was appointed: this initiative facilitated the setting up of a regional research strategy and network and would enable resources for research to be earmarked. This coincided with the drive in Western medicine for greater application of evidence based medical treatment.

A few keen general practitioners had used computers in their practices in the 1970s; numbers grew slowly during the 1980s as the technology improved and costs fell. By 1990 around 80% of practices were computerised, a figure that continued to rise as the 1990 contract bedded in and GPs acknowledged the need for effective information systems.

1991   The NHS internal market opened in April and the first wave of volunteer GP fundholders started operating. The first tranche of NHS trusts was also set up. The reform would prove to be the start of a shift from a secondary to primary care led NHS and therefore of professional power from consultants to general practice.

Doctors were worried about the effects of the internal market on clinical standards: in response, health ministers set up a Clinical Standards Advisory Group to monitor NHS standards.

The government brought in the Citizens' Charter to cover the private and public sectors. In the NHS, for instance, standards were set for the time within which patients should be seen in accident and emergency departments and how long patients should wait for operations. The charter was to lead to the later publication of hospital league tables, a controversial measure of hospitals' performances. It also declared that citizens had the "right to receive health care on the basis of clinical needs regardless of ability to pay".

The problems of London's health services had been a troublesome thread running through the NHS since 1948. The NHS outside London envied the capital's apparent financial advantages - only part altered by RAWP - yet many services in London were inadequate. Several reviews over the years had not provided an effective comprehensive solution. In 1991, William Waldegrave announced a strategic review of London's health services chaired by Sir Bernard Tomlinson, chairman of the Northern Regional Health Authority.

A *New Deal* was agreed between the Health Departments and the medical profession to reduce the workload of hard pressed hospital junior staff. Progress was made in cutting the number on call for over 72 hours a week. This, however, had a knock on effect on consultants' hours of duty and the time available for training young doctors. Increases in the number of consultant posts was not keeping pace with the targets set in the 1986 report, *Achieving a Balance*.

A Green Paper, *The Health of the Nation,* was published with the aim of producing a comprehensive health policy that crossed government departmental boundaries and shifted the emphasis from people as patients to people as consumers. The Green Paper was based on the premise that health was a product of several factors from environmental to individuals' life styles.

1992   The White Paper *The Health of the Nation* firmed up the ideas in the

1991 Green Paper. Acknowledging that governments had wider responsibilities for health other than providing a health care system, the White Paper laid down 25 specific policy targets. These included, for example, the reduction of the death rate for stroke and coronary heart disease in the under 65s by 40% by the turn of the century. No mention was made, however, of the effects of unemployment and poverty on people's health.

In April 1992 John Major led the Conservative Party to its fourth consecutive election victory. Virginia Bottomley took over as Secretary of State for Health.

Two inquiries on London's health services reported. The first, from a commission appointed by the King's Fund, accepted the case for substantial change, urging cuts in acute services and development of primary care. It criticised London hospitals for being "top heavy with doctors". The second, the government initiated Tomlinson inquiry, also called for better primary care services and proposed specially funded London Initiative Zones. The report wanted further rationalisation of hospitals and medical schools. In 1993 the Department of Health broadly accepted the Tomlinson report.

Comprising nearly 300,000 of the NHS staff in England, nurses remained by far the largest working group. Their education, clinical responsibilities and management, however, had undergone great changes since the 1960s, with the skill mix within nursing constantly being refined, nurses working more independently of doctors and the division of nursing into clinical nurses and nurse managers developing. The nursing process had replaced the more disciplinarian, care of the patient approach inherent in the Nightingale tradition. In 1992 the UKCC published guidance on the scope of professional practice and codes of professional conduct (*Guidelines for Professional Practice*). This accelerated the switch from a previously hierarchical profession to one based on professional autonomy, with nurses responsible for their own practice and competence.

In 1992-3 13% of GPs had opted for fundholding status.

The newly appointed Medical Manpower Standing Advisory Committee forecast a persisting shortage of doctors in the UK. A rising number of junior staff were having to be recruited from the European Community. This was because doctors from the Indian subcontinent and elsewhere, who had since the 1960s filled the gap between the supply of UK trained doctors and the NHS's requirements for medical staff, were facing restrictions as a result of Britain's stricter immigration rules. Such doctors were admitted only for training for a set period. Doctors from the European Community, however, had unrestricted access. The number of women medical students qualifying in the UK had steadily risen to a point where their numbers slightly exceeded that of men. Since some women graduates did not practice full time in the NHS this reduced the effective size of the medical workforce. The advisory committee proposed a rise in UK annual intake to 4,470 places, with a target of 4,970 for 2000.

The House of Commons Health Select Committee called for a change in traditional obstetric practice that all births should be in hospital. This led to a mixed expert and consumers group producing *Changing Childbirth* (in 1993), a report that recommended giving women a greater choice in where they should be delivered and by whom.

1993   The number of preregistration doctors wanting to enter general practice fell to 25%, a drop from 45% in a decade. Workloads of GPs were rising and morale was falling.

The government published its response to the Tomlinson report on London's health services. It formed a London Implementation Group and six specialty reviews. A radical framework of five administrative sectors was set up. London Iniiative Zones were established to revitalise primary care.

In April 99 more NHS trusts joined the first wave of 57 launched in April 1992. The effectiveness of trusts varied widely, some successfully expanding their services, others running into serious financial difficulties. Overall, the NHS continued to have financial problems despite extra funding earmarked for the costs of introducing reform.

The government set up a review on the future structure of health authorities.

A National Blood Authority was set up, despite some protests that this would make the transfusion service less responsive to local needs, a criticism endorsed in a daming report in 1998.

The Calman report was published. The outcome of an inquiry led by the Chief Medical Officer, Sir Kenneth Calman, its purpose was to marry up European Community requirements for specialist practice with UK arrangements in which junior doctors spent longer in training posts than their European colleagues. A complex problem, any proposals had to take account of the NHS services provided by junior staff and the balance between training and career grade status. Calman proposed a single specialist training grade and structured training requirements. After up to six years of satisfactory training a doctor would be awarded a certificate of completion of specialist training, which would make him or her eligible for a consultant post.

1994   *Doctors and their Careers*, (by Isobel Allen) was published. An expert on the medical workforce, she highlighted the problems facing women doctors. They needed flexible training and work with part-time possibilities. Junior doctors of both sexes were critical about overwork, lack of career counselling and unsatisfactory teaching methods.

Government published comparative performance guide (league tables) showing extent to which hospitals had achieved performance targets. These "league tables", seen as controversial by health professionals, were intended to help individuals and their GPs "make informed decisions" about their healthcare.

A King's Fund report, *Evaluating the NHS Reforms*, showed how hard it was to evaluate effectively the consequences of the internal market.

Government published *Health Authorities Bill* which would abolish regional health authorities - replacing them with regional outposts of the NHS Executive - and merging district health and family health services authorities to form 100 single health authorities in England. The latter would bring family practitioner services into the mainstream of NHS management. The changes were planned for 1996.

The Department of Health published the Banks report defining the responsibilities of the Department and the NHS Executive, a cause of confusion since the latter's establishment. The Executive would be responsible for both policy formulation and implementation, with the Department left with a varied collection of other responsibilities.

Between 1990-1 and 1994-5 the number of medical emergencies admitted to hospitals rose by 10%. Accident and emergency departments were finding it increasingly difficult to cope with the number of patients attending, and assaults on staff by patients were becoming a serious problem. The length of time patients stayed in hospital had been steadily shortening, with day wards increasingly used. The shortage of beds for patients needing treatment was made worse because beds were being blocked by elderly patients who though suitable for care in the community could not be transferred because of inadequate resources for community care. Implementation of the community care aspects of the 1991 legislative reforms - introduced in 1993 - was being handicapped because of resource shortages.

The government-initiated Culyer report on the funding of NHS research recommended that the diversity of funding arrangements should be replaced by a single NHS budget. A subsequent survey (1996) identified 39,000 research projects in the NHS, most of them in acute and community health trusts: £330 million went on supporting research and development.

In November leading organisations in the medical profession published *Core Values for the Medical Profession in the 21st Century*.

The Audit Commission published *Finding a Place: A Review of Mental Health Services for Adults*. It identified the main challenge as managerial rather than clinical and set out an action plan for all levels of the NHS.

1995   General practitioners were increasingly angry at their rising out of hours workload . The BMA and the government eventually in 1996 agreed contractual changes that gave GPs more discretion on whether and where they should see patients wanting attention out of normal working hours. GPs were also arguing for a new contract that covered certain "core services", and their leaders pressed the government for such a change.

NHS staff numbers had fallen by 30,000 between 1990 and 1995; 93% of the 764,000 staff in 1995 were non-medical and two thirds were directly caring for patients.

The number of GPs had risen by over 10% (mainly women) between 1985 and 1995.

The Medical (Professional Performance) Bill introduced in March. It arose from an initiative by the General Medical Council to set up a procedure for dealing with doctors whose professional performance was unsatisfactory but did not constitute serious professional misconduct.

The BMA's consultants committee published *The Consultant Charter* defining what it saw as NHS consultants' responsibilities and rights.

The government tightened up the procedures for individuals claiming incapacity benefits.

The Doctors' Tale, an Audit Commission report on the activities of hospital doctors, analysed the work of the 55,000 or so hospital doctors in England and Wales. It concluded that despite changes in health care and NHS structure doctors' working practices had "stayed much the same and are now inappropriate for the context in which they work". The commission called for better training strategies, a clearer definition of doctors' roles, annually reviewed and monitored job plans for consultants and more positive relationships between doctors and managers.

The disagreements over the future of London's health services continued. Demanding firm government action, a chairman of an earlier review of London's medical schools wrote in *The Times*: "During the past twenty years ... every attempt to reform London medicine has been defeated by vigorous rearguard action on behalf of any hospital or medical school adversely affected." The internal market had highlighted London's weaknesses and the Secretary of State, Virginia Bottomley, took some hard decisions on closures and mergers.

In July Stephen Dorrell succeeded Virginia Bottomley as Secretary of State for Health.

By the end of 1995 plans were in hand for the expenditure of £2 billion on over 50 capital schemes nationwide to make use of the government's introduction of the Private Finance Initiative into the NHS, but the plans were slow to be translated into health service real estate.

The NHS introduced a scheme, announced in 1992, to allocate every patient an individual number: this would facilitate the transmission of management and clinical data within the service. The national system was planned to be in place by 1998.

A much publicised court case - others had preceded it - occurred over the right of the NHS to withhold treatment from a patient when the health authority believed that its cost effectiveness was unproved. In this instance the health authority lost, but the case highlighted the problem of treatment priorities, a subject being widely debated by health professionals, managers, politicians and the media. Decisions long made "covertly" by clinicians on rationing treatments were now being forced into the open by the financial pressure of the internal market.

The Royal College of Physicians published *Setting priorities in the NHS*; this was followed up by a *BMJ* leading article in June calling on the government to take a lead on rationing care.

Several cases of psychiatric patients with serious illness living in the community with inadequate supervision and becoming a danger to themselves and the public led to the Mental Health (Patients in the Community) Act 1995. This allowed authorised supervisors to take such patients to hospital if they believed this to be necessary. Solution of this serious sociomedical problem continued to be handicapped by a lack of suitable facilities and resources.

To combat burgeoning bureaucracy in NHS the Department of Health published *Patients not Paper*. It planned to start implementing the 65 recommendations in December.

The Medical (Professional Performance) Act 1995 amended the 1993 Act to include new professional performance procedures (controlled by GMC) to tackle poorly performing doctors. In parallel, the government issued guidance *Maintaining Medical Excellence*.

Government published *Acting on Complaints* aimed at streamlining and strengthening procedures for patients to complain about NHS services.

1996   NHS trust chief executives warned Stephen Dorrell, Secretary of

State for Health, that financial meltdown in the NHS was a possibility because of rising demands, rising management costs and perverse incentives in the internal market. The BMA appealed to the Prime Minister to tackle the crisis in underfunding.

The Pharmaceutical Price Regulation Scheme in a report to Parliament claimed that in 1995 it had saved £90m compared to the NHS's 1994 drug bill.

Parliament's Public Accounts Committee reported in *Clinical Audit in England* 86% participation by GPs and 83% by hospital doctors but warned that it was hard to determine the impact of audit on patient care.

In 1993 the responsibility for funding the education of nurses was transferred to trust and health authorities (acting in groups) which meant that numbers trained were based more on available finance than on clinical requirements. Unrest among nurses over poor pay - a long running feature of the NHS - and increasing workloads led to a serious shortage of nurses and wastage rates of 20%. Hospitals became increasingly reliant on agency nurses.

In a consultation document the NHS Executive proposed a radical overhaul in the funding of medical education based on a system of local purchasing.

The government published three White Papers on the NHS. *Choice and Opportunity* and *Primary Care: delivering the future* dealt with primary care. The aim was to widen the responsibilities of this sector and make its operation more flexible. The second document came out in December and among several proposals were minimum vocational training standards, introduction of salaried GPs, more money for research and development and an extension of nurse prescribing. *A Service with Ambitions* was the third White Paper: it reaffirmed Britain's commitment to a state funded health service of steadily rising quality available to all citizens on the basis of clinical need regardless of ability to pay. The government repeated its commitment to raise health funding in real terms.

General practitioners' annual conference overwhelmingly supported the principal of defined core services in general medical services and demanded a new contract based on these.

A large group of national organisations, including some representing doctors, nurses, social services, health authorities and trusts, as well as Age Concern, recommended nationally defined, minimum levels of long term care for all, free at the point of delivery.

1997 An official report in January showed that at least 8,000 junior hospital doctors were still working more than 72 hours a week.

Also in January, the BMA claimed that many NHS trusts would start the financial year with substantial deficits. The National Association of Health Authorities and Trusts had previously warned that the NHS needed an extra £200m for 1996-7.

The NHS (Primary Care) Act, passed in March, would, from April 1998, allow NHS trusts and GPs to take part in pilot schemes to provide personal medical services on a salaried basis or using other financial managements. The Act contained other provisions (see 1996 White Papers).

In May the Labour Party won the general election with a landslide majority; the NHS had been an important issue in the campaign. Frank Dobson became Secretary of State for Health and Tessa Jowell public health minister, a new post.

In July the new government promised an extra £1.26bn for the NHS from April 1998, and in October it announced an extra £300m - £30m of it from efficiency savings - to boost NHS patient care during the forthcoming winter. (These figures should be seen in the context of estimated gross NHS spending in the UK for 1997-8 of over £44bn - 5.6% of the gross domestic product). Later in the year health ministers announced emergency steps to ease winter pressures by giving trusts greater flexibility in their budgeting processes.

The Chancellor, Gordon Brown, announced that the Treasury's fundamental review of public spending would look for new ways of funding the NHS.

The Audit Commission recommended a reduction in specialists' participation in routine antenatal care. Its report, *First Class Delivery: improving maternity services in England and Wales*, pointed out the wide variations in the numbers of medical interventions during pregnancy and labour, prompting a call to avoid unnecessary interventions.

Health authorities started piloting a new way of increasing the public's input into NHS decision making by organising citizen's juries on key local issues.

White Paper, *The New NHS*, published in December, was the Labour Government's first major presentation of its health policy. The aim was to renew the NHS as a one nation health service more closely integrated with social care. The document proposed phasing out the internal market, including GP fundholding. The government promised a Commission for Health Improvement, a National Institute of Clinical Excellence, new ways of measuring trusts' efficiency, the setting up of primary care groups to link GPs and community nurses in commissioning health care and better feedback from patients and users.

Designed to Care, a White Paper published simultaneously with *The New NHS*, contained plans for the NHS in Scotland. The agenda of radical reform of the internal market was similar to that for England. The new Scottish Parliament, however, would assume responsibility for the reformed NHS. (Plans for Wales and Northern Ireland were due to be announced in 1998.)

The government promised a revised Patients' Charter, emphasising patients' responsibilities to the NHS.

The NHS Executive published *Clinical Guidelines: using clinical guidelines to improve patient care within the NHS*.

Mid-year the National Audit Office reported that 36 out of 100 health authorities had forecast deficits of over £1m at the end of 1996-7, double the previous year's number; 168 of 433 trusts were in financial trouble. After the general election Department of Health briefings of ministers had forecast that projected NHS funding for the next two years was totally inadequate.

Government announced (another) independent review of London's health services; Sir Leslie Turnberg, president of Royal College of Physicians would chair it.

Government introduced new health strategy to take account of link between poverty and health and to encourage an integrated

214

approach. All government policies would be evaluated for potential impact on the nation's health. Sir Donald Acheson (a former Chief Medical Officer) appointed to chair an independent review of health inequalities.

Secretary of State for Health promised revised government approach to NHS staff's pay aimed at "a combination of national pay determination with appropriate local flexibility".

Official figures showed that the number of GP trainees had fallen by 21% between 1986 and 1996 but that the total number of GPs had risen by 9% to nearly 29,000, 14% of whom worked part time and 32% of whom were women. On average, each GP had 8% fewer patients on his or her list in 1996 than in 1986.

Laing's Review of Private Health Care 1997, reported that spending on private medical insurance rose by 10% in 1996 to £1.8bn. NHS facilities had attracted 15% of private patients activity. Fees paid to doctors at around £650m meant that the 17,500 NHS consultants who did private practice received an annual average *gross* revenue of £37,500 from this source.

In *The Coming of Age* the Audit Commission urged the NHS and social services to collaborate to improve care for older people with the emphasis shifted to caring for people at home.

The government outlawed "gagging clauses" in NHS staff's employment contracts so that staff could speak their minds on genuine concerns about NHS or patient care without fear of victimisation.

1998   As the UK entered its six months presidency of the European Union, the government outlined its health policy aims for the EU. These included a ban on tobacco advertising, a network for communicable disease surveillance and effective EU action for improving public health.

In a White Paper, *The Food Standards Agency: a formula for change*, the government announced that the health departments would take over responsibility for food from the Ministry of Agriculture and Fisheries. The proposed Food Standards Agency, set to start work in 1999, would protect consumers' interests. The public had lost

215

confidence in the existing arrangements after the prolonged crisis - which started in 1986 - over the health implications of the bovine spongiform encephalopathy (BSE) epidemic, a sharply rising incidence of food poisoning in the population and serious, widely publicised, outbreaks of infection caused by *Escherichia coli* contamination of meat.

NHS Wales: putting patients first, a White Paper on changes to the NHS in Wales, planned for a minimum of 22 local health groups, containing GPs, pharmacists, nurses, dentists and other professionals, which would take responsibility of commissioning health services. The changes proposed were broadly similar to those for England and Scotland and the new Welsh Assembly would have a pivotal role in health policy.

A 1997 report showing NHS prescription fraud was costing £100m annually prompted the health departments to launch a new drive to prevent fraud by health professionals and patients.

The Royal College of Nursing warned of the worst recruitment crisis in NHS nursing for 25 years. The number of entrants was at its lowest ever level and the health service was short of over 8,000 full time nurses, with standards of patient care at risk. A key factor was poor pay, according to the RCN.

An independent report stated that NHS trusts made almost £250m in 1996-7 by treating private patients, a rise of 14% on the previous year. The sum, however, represented on average barely 1% of trusts' incomes from their core activities, though for specialist trusts the average figure was nearly 7%.

The government announced the launch of six health action zones which would focus the joint efforts of NHS bodies and local authorities on reducing health inequalities. Eleven areas of England covering six million people were selected for this initiative.

The Nuffield Trust published *Improving the Health of the NHS Workforce*, a report calling on health ministers to initiate a ten point plan to tackle the high burden of ill health among NHS staff. The report pointed out that 27% of healthcare staff reported high levels of psychological disturbance. The figure was 18% in the general working population.

'*New Ambitions for our country: A New Contract for Welfare*' was published. A Green Paper outlining the broad sweep of the government's plans for reforming Britain's Welfare State, it was based around the principle of "empowerment not dependency" and was tied in with the drive to get people off benefits into work. If successful, it could contribute to reducing inequalities within the population and so help to relieve the rising demands on the NHS, which, on its 50th birthday, was experiencing increasing strain.

The government announced that waiting lists for hospitals admission stood at 1,420,000 - a rise of 100,000 in England alone sine May 1997 - and were still rising. Secretary of state Frank Dobson announced that £320 million of the extra funds earmarked for the NHS in the March budget would go directly to cutting waiting lists by 100,000 by March 1999 (Scotland and Wales had targets of 4,000 and 2,000). He urged NHS trusts and managers to meet new targets set by the government, including the elimination of waiting times of 18 months.

Index